The Reign of Error

The Reign of Error

Psychiatry, Authority, and Law

Lee Coleman, M.D.

Beacon Press *Boston*

Copyright © 1984 by Lee Coleman

Beacon Press books are published under the auspices
of the Unitarian Universalist Association
of Congregations in North America,
25 Beacon Street, Boston, Massachusetts 02108

Published simultaneously in Canada by
Fitzhenry & Whiteside Limited, Toronto

Library of Congress Cataloging in Publication Data

Coleman, Lee, 1938–
   The reign of error.

   Bibliography: p.
   Includes index.
   1. Forensic psychiatry—United States. 2. Insanity—
Jurisprudence—United States. 3. Criminal liability—
United States. I. Title.
KF8922.C64   1984   614′.1   83-71943
ISBN 0-8070-0481-2

Acknowledgments

I am deeply grateful for the help I received from a number of persons, without whom this book might still be in my head and not on paper. John Schonenberg and Bob Meinsma spent many hours in legal libraries and medical libraries, digging out reference materials. Sarah Leslie and Marcy Holtz transformed my sometimes barely readable pages into typed manuscript.

Literary agent Fred Hill had faith in my message from the beginning yet would not allow me to be satisfied with less than my best. Grant Morris read portions of the manuscript and made useful suggestions. Free-lance editor Marilyn Landau was of immense help in shaping an unwieldy manuscript into what is, I hope, a clear and cogent treatment of my subject. Her stamp on this book is profound.

I wish to thank, in addition, senior editor Marie Cantlon, managing editor Jeff Smith, and the staff at Beacon Press for their outstanding editorial assistance and for their support of this book. Susan Oleksiw and Leonard Frank gave me first-rate editorial help in the final stages.

Finally, my wife and children offered me the support needed to carry on with the task of summarizing a decade of work.

CONTENTS

Introduction

Every year more than a million American citizens are forced to enter mental hospitals and undergo dangerous psychiatric treatments they have never agreed to.[1] And every year thousands of citizens accused of crimes though not convicted by a court are confined in mental institutions.[2] Abuses such as these occur because psychiatrists wield the state-given power to decide what is good for another person.

Similarly, nonviolent lawbreakers who stand trial and are then sentenced to prison may serve additional years because a psychiatrist has labeled them dangerous. At the same time violent murderers and rapists may be released from prison after only a few months, because a psychiatrist declares them to be no longer dangerous.

The opinion of a psychiatrist may determine the final outcome in the matter of wills, contracts, adoptions, child custody, hirings, firings, probation, and parole. Psychiatrists may influence whether a person is allowed to drive a car, join or leave the military, spend money, sue or be sued, and vote. Yet psychiatrists have no valid scientific tools or expertise to justify their legal power. Indeed, while psychotherapy may help emotionally troubled persons, state-imposed psychiatry helps neither the patients nor society in general. If society is ever to deal effectively with the problems of deviant behavior, violence, and criminal responsibility it now places on psychiatrists' shoulders, this power must be completely abolished.

I have not always held this view. At the beginning of my career as a psychiatrist, I was convinced, along with most other psychiatrists, that in certain situations psychiatrists were obligated to apply their skills and to prescribe treatments. Society needed us, for example, to take care of the mentally disordered if they were dangerous, suicidal, or unable to cope, even if they did not want our help. Psychiatrists were also needed to testify in court: In what other way could a judge or jury learn enough about a person's mental state to make a valid decision? This was true whether the case involved legal insanity, alleged psychic trauma from an automobile accident, or potentially dangerous mental illness. In addition, society needed us to rehabilitate adult and juvenile prisoners, because crime supposedly stemmed from mental disturbance. And prisons, finally, needed us to determine which inmates were cured and thus ready for release. Since we were essential to society in all these situations, lawmakers had no apparent choice except to give psychiatrists the legal power to do whatever they thought necessary.

I once agreed with this position, but I now consider it outmoded and dangerous. My experiences as a psychiatrist tell me that psychiatry should be stripped of its state-given powers for two main reasons. First, psychiatrists do not have the tools that society thinks they have. They have no special way of predicting who will commit a criminal act or of determining when a criminal is cured of antisocial tendencies. They have no tests to determine a person's innermost thoughts, even though the courts assume they do. Second, problems associated with psychiatric power are really ethical and political considerations rather than scientific or medical ones. Thus, when a psychiatrist uses legal authority to involuntarily hospitalize a person whose behavior is disturbing, the psychiatrist is acting more on behalf of the community than on behalf of the patient. Similarly, when a psychiatrist testifies on legal insanity, medical language is used to present opinions on the legal and ethical question of criminal responsibility. Such language may not truly help our courts, but it certainly helps psychiatry.

For unlike other mental health professionals, psychiatrists are medical doctors. The person choosing a career in psychiatry must complete medical school, an internship, and a psychiatric residency of three years. As physicians, psychiatrists are bound to approach problems (even nonmedical ones like criminal responsibility) from a medical perspective.

Because of this medical training, society grants certain privileges and responsibilities to the psychiatrist. Society gives him or her the final say in mental hospital settings, and allows the psychiatrist, rather than other mental health professionals, to prescribe medications. For society assumes that the psychiatrist, like any other medical doctor, can apply certain tests to accurately diagnose mental diseases and then draw on known medical treatments for specific illnesses. In response to these expectations, psychiatrists do apply "tests" and they do "diagnose" their patients' problems—that is, they do pick a diagnostic term from a catalog of officially sanctioned labels and they do prescribe treatments that other psychotherapists may not prescribe.

Medical doctors have traditionally been assigned the control and care of mentally deviant persons. For hundreds of years, doctors known as alienists headed asylums for the mentally disordered. Because alienists were physicians, society expected them to apply physical treatments to asylum inmates. And so they did.

Society today expects the same type of service from its psychiatrists. More and more people have accepted psychiatry's claim that major mental disorder is a sign of a disordered brain and thus a medical problem. Although some psychiatrists still see mental disorder as a sign of a troubled life rather than a troubled brain, psychiatrists are being trained to prescribe medications for an ostensibly physical problem, as other medical doctors do. This position is justified only in a few selected situations where behavioral or mental symptoms might indeed be the result of medical conditions. These include chemical or hormonal imbalances, infections, and brain tumors. In these circumstances, it is important, even critical, that the attending therapist be able to recognize the underlying medical problem. Similarly, in surgical and medical cases and in consultations concerning possible use of psychoactive drugs, it is important that the attending therapist have medical knowledge.

Because contemporary society assumes that the medical trappings of psychiatry make it a science, society also assumes that psychiatry deserves to wield legal power in mental hospitals, in courts, and in prisons. In this book I will refute that assumption: I will show that psychiatry does not deserve the legal power it has been given, that, indeed, psychiatry is not a science. Rather, psychiatry is an art. As a psychotherapist in private practice, I daily see how the art of the therapeutic relationship can help. But helping people who seek out therapy is one thing; using legal power to control the lives of such persons is quite another. For this reason alone psychiatry shorn of all legal power would offer more effective and meaningful help to those who ask for it and therefore to society as a whole.

The views expressed here about my own profession developed gradually over several years. In 1971 I moved with my family to California after completing my training at the University of Colorado Medical Center and serving two years as a staff psychiatrist at the U.S. Air Force Academy. I was ready to begin my career as a psychiatrist in a San Francisco Bay Area clinic. On August 21, 1971, one month after I began my new job, a prisoner named George Jackson was killed in San Quentin prison.

Considered a leader by militant black convicts, Jackson had been accused months earlier, along with two other black convicts, of killing a guard at Soledad prison. This killing had taken place just hours after a grand jury had failed to indict another guard for shooting and killing three unarmed black prisoners during a fight with whites. Although I did not know it at the time, this event opened to me my new work: the relationship between psychiatry and the state.

Interested in these explosive developments, I began to read Jackson's book, *Soledad Brother*.[3] This very moving book offered a collection of letters Jackson had written to his attorney Fay Stender, during Jackson's ten years' confinement for robbery of a liquor store. From these letters I learned that the parole board could deny a man his freedom for merely subjective reasons.

Jackson described his numerous appearances before the parole board, known then as the Adult Authority. He felt that the board, in deciding when to release him from a one-year-to-life sentence, paid more attention to his attitude than to his crime. He believed that because he was a political militant and unwilling to passively accept what he considered unjust prison conditions, the board repeatedly denied him parole. Years earlier, he noted, they had released more passive prisoners who had committed far more serious crimes. Feeling that the board hearings were a sham, Jackson burned with a sense of injustice.

Based on a psychological model of crime and prisons, the one-year-to-life sentence promised that release would come as soon as the prisoner's "treatment" was complete. Yet the uncertainty and potential injustice the sentence implied was beginning to look to me like brutalizing punishment. This was a far cry, I told myself, from what psychiatrist Karl Menninger had promised in *The Crime of Punishment*, a book that summarized a generation of liberal thinking about prisons and one that I had accepted completely during my psychiatry training.[4]

I was angry at myself for having been duped and then began to feel that as a psychiatrist I might be able to help raise a few questions about indeterminate sentencing policies. I contacted an organization called the Committee for Prisoner Humanity and Justice, and through them I began to learn more about the role of psychiatry in prisons and parole decisions.

As my criticism of the parole process grew and became known in the San Francisco Bay Area, a few attorneys asked me to testify before or write reports to parole boards. In these reports I pointed out, first, that psychiatrists had no special way to tell when a prisoner was ready for release and, second, that prison treatment programs were accomplishing nothing positive.

In 1975 another public event influenced my work: the trial of Patricia Hearst. Hearst had been photographed with members of the Symbionese Liberation Army while they robbed San Francisco's Hibernia Bank. The films showed her waving a machine gun and cursing at terrified bank customers. Before the trial started, defense attorney F. Lee Bailey asked for a hearing to determine whether Hearst was competent to stand trial. It was a legal ploy, of course, since nothing indicated she was out of touch with reality.

At this point law professor George Alexander and I decided to speak out about psychiatry's inability to determine competence for trial. Both of us were convinced that psychiatrists had no special skills in this area; indeed, as dean of the Santa Clara University School of Law, Alexander spoke as an acknowledged expert on the problems of psychiatric testimony. We held a press conference, presented our views, received little coverage for our impassioned pleas, and went back to work at our respective tasks, practicing psychiatrist and academic dean.

The press conference, however, did have some repercussions. Two months later I received a call from the district attorney in Sacramento. He asked if I would be willing to testify, at an upcoming trial, on legal insanity, but not about what the accused person, a man in his twenties, was supposedly thinking when he committed the crime, which is what psychiatrists ordinarily do in criminal trials. Rather he wanted me to state again what I had stated at the earlier press conference on the Hearst case: Psychiatrists do not have tests to measure a person's mind. I agreed to testify.

A few weeks later I received another request, but this time it came from the public defender. The state had alleged that his client, a woman in her fifties, could not care for herself because of mental disorder, and the state was therefore threatening to take control of her life. Now it was the district attorney who was hiring psychiatrists to testify against the woman, and the defense attorney who was trying to nullify their comments. Once again I agreed to testify, but only on the condition that I would not have to speak about the state of her mind; rather I would testify about the state of psychiatry. I would testify that psychiatrists' tools were not any better than those available to lay persons to determine if this woman could care for herself. The practical facts of her case, I told the jury, would better guide them to a correct decision than any psychiatric evaluation of her mental state.

Since those two trials I have testified in over one hundred and thirty criminal and civil trials around the country, countering the authority of psychiatrists or psychologists hired by one side or the other. In each case I try to educate the judge or jury about why the opinions produced by these professionals have no scientific merit, that indeed no psychiatrist or psychologist can ever determine what a person was thinking at any time in the past, or what a person will do in the future. During these trials I offer no opinion about anyone's state of mind, and instead urge the court to base its decision on the facts of the case. Factual evidence, rather than psychiatric speculation, provides the most valid grounds on which to base a decision. There is no better way to determine whether or not a defendant had criminal intent, or whether a mental patient is competent, or whether an automobile accident caused psychological injury.

My work in these trials, along with my work in mental hospitals and prisons, has given me access to much information that is generally restricted. Because this secrecy helps hide the truth from the public—the truth that psychiatrists do not really possess the expertise they claim—I want to share this information with you and let you decide what role psychiatry should play in our society.

When people understand what psychiatrists really do with the legal power society gives them, people will gradually insist on new laws that annul this power.

I see no grand conspiracies or villains among psychiatrists. We are all heirs to a tradition that hems us in. We all have relied on psychiatry for so many decades that we feel naked without its protective garb. And when I suggest that we strip this garb away, I do not mean to imply that society's problems will disappear. The problems we now expect psychiatrists to solve will remain, serious and complex. But only when we stop relying on psychiatry to solve problems it cannot solve will we be free to turn our attention to alternative—and ultimately more effective—approaches. Only when psychiatrists stop forcing their aid on unwilling patients, stop making courtroom pronouncements, and stop playing an unwarranted role in shaping social policies will we be free to find our way toward policies that offer more hope for us all.

The Reign of Error

CHAPTER 1

THE REIGN OF ERROR

When the Chicago police started to arrest Robert Friedman for panhandling in front of a downtown bus station on August 2, 1975, he pleaded, "Don't take me in. I'm not broke. I didn't know this was a crime." He opened his briefcase and revealed to the officers $24,087 in small bills. "A few days later," according to a report by the Associated Press, "he was committed to a mental institution by a judge who said he was protecting Friedman from thugs who might be after his cash."

Thugs never got Friedman's cash, but psychiatry did. He was forced to pay for his incarceration in a psychiatric hospital, and even had to pay the fees for the lawyer who convinced the judge to lock him up. Twelve thousand dollars later, Friedman was finally able to get help from DePaul University law professor Edward J. Benett, who commented, "He was committed on the possibility that he would be mugged, beaten and robbed, and instead he's locked up, filled with drugs and his money is taken gradually instead of in one clean sweep."[1]

This is an example of what I call psychiatry's reign of error. I mean by this the exercise of the vast power that our society grants psychiatry and that psychiatry so readily accepts. The immense legal power given to psychiatry is based on faith, not reason. Society assumes that during their training psychiatrists are taught to do all of the things we have come to expect of them. This is a natural assumption. During training psychiatrists get plenty of practice doing psychotherapy. They also learn about psychoactive

1

drugs and the body's reaction to them. They learn about family relationships, child development, and group therapy. They gain experience offering consultation to medical patients, school personnel, and community agencies. They learn how some medical disorders may lead to mental dysfunction.

Yet society also expects psychiatrists to go farther—to deal with the ethical and legal issues surrounding deviant behavior, criminal responsibility, public safety. In the process we overlook that psychiatrists are not trained to be expert or scientific in these matters.

The essence of science is objectivity and reliability. In science, personal opinion is replaced by methods of data collection that are replicable. While medicine has many methods of objective data collection, psychiatry's methods rely on subjective impressions.

Psychiatry's "Examinations"

Psychiatrists encourage the view that psychiatry rests on a scientific basis because medical authority confers leadership in the mental health professions. The use of medical language gives to the art of psychiatry an undeserved scientific status. Conversation with a psychiatrist, for example, is called a clinical examination. The result of this conversation is not a personal opinion but a diagnosis.

Let us consider, for example, the "mental status examination." According to a standard textbook, the examination allows a psychiatrist "to obtain a precise picture of the patient's emotional status and mental capacity and functioning."[2] How is this "precise" picture obtained? By observing appearance, behavior, mood, content of speech, and ideas. The psychiatrist also asks about current events and has the person do simple arithmetic. In addition, the patient is asked to interpret proverbs on the theory that the answers will tell the psychiatrist whether the patient is brain injured or psychotic.

Asking questions is one thing; interpreting the answers is quite another. Cultural, linguistic, and educational factors may influence virtually every question and answer. If the person is being treated involuntarily, he or she may express resentment by giving inadequate or hostile answers. Such responses are often interpreted as signs of mental disorder.

Can we then say that a psychiatric interview equals a bona fide examination of the type we expect from a physician? The fact that several psychiatrists frequently reach different conclusions about the same patient tells us that these interviews are not strictly scientific. Rather they are merely a period of discussion and observation through which one person (the psychiatrist) tries to decide what he or she thinks of the other (the patient). Information may be gathered, but the *interpretation* is intensely subjective. The psychiatrist's personality, his or her school of thought, the setting of the interview—all these things influence the conclusions in ways that are hidden rather than explicit and are impossible to measure.

That psychiatry's conversations and observations are subjective does not imply that nothing valuable may result. Capable psychiatrists may use their impressions and their observations wisely, to offer real help to their patients. The error made here is the assumption that these conversations lead to *scientific* results; they do not. They give the perceptive psychiatrist an understanding of another human being, but no data to use in answering ethical or legal questions.

Psychology's "Tests"

Psychological tests rely more heavily on numbers and graphs, but the results are no more scientific.[3] If anything, the mischief may be even more pronounced. Whereas psychiatrists make their opinions appear scientific through the use of medical language, psychologists make their opinions appear scientific through the use of charts and statistics. But regardless of the mode of presenting the results, the psychologists, just as much as psychiatrists, must *interpret* the patient's test responses, and this act of interpretation is inherently subjective. Again, physicians must interpret test results, but they begin with data that are inherently different from the data of psychology. A borderline thyroid hormone level may be open to interpretation, but the amount of thyroid hormone is beyond question. A sputum culture that produces tuberculosis organisms will indicate the correct diagnosis regardless of the physician's political leanings or personality. The same cannot be said for the data of psychology.

One of the clearest examples of subjectivity masquerading as science in the field of psychological testing is the widespread use of computers to score the answers to a personality questionnaire such as the Minnesota Multiphasic Personality Inventory (MMPI). The patient takes a true-false examination and the answers are fed into a computer that has been programmed to interpret the choices. The answers are graphed and appear to give objective measures of personality. But these graphs hide the fact that someone has previously decided what is a normal response and what is an abnormal response to each question. The computer sorts and catalogs the answers and prints out predigested conclusions, but the conclusions are only worth as much as the initial judgments fed into the computer.[4]

Such pseudoscience also prevails with the Rorschach test. A person is asked to interpret a standard series of cards, each of which contains an inkblot. The response to each card becomes the basis for the psychologist's evaluation of the patient's mental state. Once again, the responses are compared with alleged normal and abnormal responses determined by the test's designer. Since the designer's interpretation of possible responses rested on his personal views rather than empirical tests, the scoring of all later patients' responses must also be subjective.[5]

Because psychologists couch their findings in scientific terms, these "tests" can easily be manipulated for any number of purposes. For example, psychologists' numbers and profiles have been used to discredit whole groups of people: Biased IQ tests have been used to support negative evaluations of blacks and other minorities.[6] The error here is to regard the "test" results as definitive. The "tests" of psychology depend on the subjective interpretation of the practitioner and are useful only as an adjunct to the clinical practice of psychiatry or psychology. Like psychiatry, psychology has no procedure to obtain objective findings.

Our Faith in Tests and Labels

How did we come to place great faith in mental health "tests"? In part we trust the practitioners of psychiatry and psychology because they are an extension of a field of science that has achieved what seems to many to be a series of miracles. Beginning around the turn of the century, physicians were able to look at a blood or sputum sample under a microscope and identify the organisms found in it; soon they could identify those that caused infectious diseases. After that came X-rays, chemotherapeutic agents, and immunizations. In a growing number of ways doctors could measure the body's functioning, make the proper diagnosis, and then treat the illness. Improved sanitation probably did even more to reduce mortality rates.[7] But there is no denying the impact of medical developments like vaccination and antibiotics. Spawned by medicine, psychology and psychiatry naturally set out to achieve the same sort of breakthroughs: These disciplines expected to perform miracles of their own.[8] If doctors could test for and cure tuberculosis or typhoid, why couldn't psychiatrists and psychologists attack the other "ills" of society, like crime, poverty, and mental disorder, by developing tests and cures of their own? Furthermore, to undertake a test was to prove one's membership in the field of medical science.

"Tests" soon abounded, couched in the language of biology and medicine and claiming to scientifically measure human behavior. By the 1920s, psychological testing was even hailed as the way to decide who was fit to immigrate to America.[9] And today we are surrounded by tests that claim to measure everything from personality to job suitability.

Social and legal custom now dictates that mental health professionals offer answers, in a wide variety of legal forums, in a manner that conveys the sense of expertise. Psychiatrists and psychologists, therefore, offer their "expert" advice even as more persons in the academic community become convinced that neither psychiatry's "examinations" nor psychology's "tests" are scientific measuring devices.[10]

Predicting Dangerousness

The legally sanctioned prediction of dangerousness illustrates the dilemmas associated with psychiatric authority. In courtrooms, mental hospitals, and prisons, crucial decisions affecting freedom or confinement, and sometimes life or death, are being made, or at least strongly influenced, by psychiatrists. For decades it was assumed that a psychiatrist could predict dangerous behavior at least as well as other doctors could prognosticate about medical illness. Finally, in the 1960s and 1970s, research studies demonstrated conclusively that psychiatric predictions of dangerousness were no better than flipping a coin.[11] In fact they were worse, because a coin flip at least is based on chance. Psychiatric predictions, the studies showed, were not only unscientific but also based on hidden, personal factors that often led to injustice.

Henry Steadman of New York's Mental Health Research Unit studied what factors lead a psychiatrist to label certain prison inmates as dangerous and others as safe.[12] He found that the psychiatrists were basing their predictions on the inmates' race, age, and type of prior offense. This meant that the psychiatrist was responding to emotions that were strictly unscientific. Young and black offenders guilty of the most serious offenses were most often the ones predicted to be dangerous. If indeed this group could be shown to be statistically the most prone to future criminality, one might argue for differential treatment. (There is, of course, the problem of the Constitution's prohibition against this sort of scheme.) But certainly this policy could not be said to rely on an "examination" of each prisoner. Steadman concluded that the psychiatrist was acting as a "conservative agent of social policy."

The research by Steadman and many others is consistent with my own impressions gained from reading hundreds of reports in which a prisoner or mental patient is proclaimed to be dangerous. The psychiatrist cites a variety of reasons for this conclusion, but in fact has no real tests to call upon. If such tests existed, they would be applied and the literature would not report the total unreliability of these predictions.

In addition to the factors mentioned by Steadman, psychiatric predictions of dangerousness are based on the psychiatrist's desire to "play it safe." If a prisoner or mental patient is released by a psychiatrist and later commits a crime, perhaps injuring or killing someone, it will be acknowledged that the psychiatrist made a terrible mistake. The psychiatrist may also worry that a victim or the victim's relative may be angry enough to bring a lawsuit. But the psychiatrist can easily avoid all this: After examining the person, the psychiatrist can simply conclude that the patient or prisoner is dangerous and must remain in custody. After this decision, possible violent behavior in the community is no longer a worry.

John Monahan, a leading investigator of predictions of dangerousness, is one of many researchers who have arrived at this conclusion. In explaining what he calls the "psychological factors involved in the overprediction of violence," he writes of the "differential consequences to the predictor."

If one overpredicts violence, the result is that individuals are incarcerated needlessly. While an unfortunate and, indeed, unjust situation, it is not likely to have significant public ramifications for the individual responsible for the overprediction. But consider the consequences for the predictor of violence should he err in the other direction—*under*prediction. The correctional officer or mental health professional who predicts that a given individual will not commit a dangerous act is subject to severe unpleasantness should that act actually occur. Often he will be informed of its consequences in the headlines ("Freed Mental Patient Murders Mother") and he or his superiors will spend many subsequent days fielding reporters' questions about his professional incompetence and his institution's laxity . . . Given the drastically differential consequences of overprediction and underprediction for the individual responsible for making the judgment, it is not surprising that he should choose to "play it safe" and err on the conservative side.[13]

Despite the tests, the interpretations, the procedures, psychiatrists make their judgments on the basis of personal values.

Determining Criminal Intent

Society also assigns to the psychiatrist the task of determining criminal responsibility. The psychiatrist may not make the final, official decision, but his or her influence is often crucial and frequently unchallenged by judges or other officials.

To make this type of determination, the psychiatrist looks backward to reconstruct the accused's state of mind during a crime rather than forward to predict potential dangerousness. Since psychiatrists have no special tests for this assignment and can only use the methodology I have already discussed—conversation, questions, observations—they inevitably present medical "findings" that are really inferences and guesses. This would be obvious to any lay person present during the "examination" of the accused, but lay people rarely if ever see this interview.

For instance, when asked by the psychiatrist to describe what happened during a crime, the accused person may reply, "I can't remember." As often as not, the psychiatrist then reports to the court that the accused suffers *amnesia* for the events of the crime, even though there is no medical reason for any loss of memory. Typically, the psychiatrist explains the amnesia by saying that the defendant went into a "dissociative state" at the moment of the crime. In ordinary language, this means that the defendant was just not himself, that he flipped into an altered state of consciousness, committed the crime, and then returned to normal, with no recollection of what happened. Or, the psychiatrist might contend that the accused lost his memory because a "brief psychosis" took over just before the crime. Let me illustrate with a recent case.[14]

"George Chapman" was smuggling gold into the country for an older man, "Albert Reed." Chapman was to receive 6 percent of the take for transferring the shipments and handling the banking. Reed discovered that Chapman was stealing from him, so he arranged a meeting at the local airport. After a few moments of conversation in a car, Chapman shot Reed as well as his female companion. She died, but Reed, though wounded, managed to escape from the car and tried to run for safety. Chapman followed, and four blocks away fired five more shots into him. Witnesses also reported seeing him kick Reed, yelling, "You son of a bitch." Chapman then ran away, but first threw the empty gun under a parked car.

Months later, after both legal insanity and diminished capacity defenses were entered by his lawyer, Chapman was interviewed by several psychiatrists and psychologists.

He claimed that Reed was the one who brought the gun and that he (Chapman) had taken it away from him. Why, then, did Chapman kill Reed's companion, chase after him, fire five bullets into him, and then kick and curse him? Chapman's initial response to these questions was that he could remember only the sound of the gun going off in the car. He later told the psychiatrist, however, that he could remember only "grabbing for the gun and a struggle ensuing."

If the psychiatrist had a special way to get inside Chapman's mind, now was the time to do so. Let us look at the psychiatrist's report on Chapman to the court:

> He describes his feelings at the time of his reaching for the gun and ensuing struggle as being a mixture of overwhelming fear, anxiety, rage, and sorrow. He says that he does, however, remember firing at Mr. Reed as the latter was leaving the car. Despite repeated attempts on my part, he was unable to describe his feelings in greater detail, saying that they were all mixed up at the time. He was also not certain as to the reason why the feelings were so intense and mixed up in the face of Mr. Reed's pointing the gun at him. At the same time, he repeatedly talks about his experiences in a way that would indicate considerable confusion on his part at the time.

An interesting explanation, perhaps, but the court wants to know whether Chapman had "criminal intent" at the moment he shot Reed. In this case, the court was told by the psychiatrist that "Mr. Chapman was very briefly in a psychotic state as a result of the intensity and severity of the stress." It was a case of temporary insanity.

The defense also brought in a psychologist, who was certainly determined to do a thorough job: He gave Chapman a total of eleven different tests. How much scientific evidence did these tests bring to bear on the question at hand: Did Chapman know what he was doing? Was his "memory loss" real or fake? Along with other tests, Chapman was shown a cartoon depicting three persons arguing over a comic book. His interpretation of this cartoon was considered by the psychologist to be "very confused, very ambivalent, very disorganized. He was utterly incapable of perceiving the social situation realistically, thinking clearly or responding appropriately." The psychologist then claimed that this cartoon scene "closely resembled the social situation at the scene of the shooting—three people concerned with the possession of a prized object (money)." He concluded that Chapman's test response "was a close approximation of his mental state at the time of the shooting." In other words, since Chapman gave an offbeat interpretation of the cartoon, he must have been in a state of "total disintegration" when he shot and killed Reed. Chapman was, the psychologist stated,

> probably not responsible for the criminal charge . . . because he was clearly experiencing a significant degree of diminished capacity as a result of mental disorder (psychotic reaction) and he therefore lacked substantial capacity to conform his conduct to the requirements of the law.

Once again, it was a case of "temporary insanity." This time the diagnosis was based on a cartoon rather than assumed amnesia.

When the prosecution presented its rebuttal, I was called to testify. As always, I pointed out to the jury that psychiatrists can only do what the jury can do—listen to the defendant's story and decide what to believe and what not to believe. The jury had not received an "expert" reconstruction from the defense psychiatrist, but rather a subjective interpretation and perhaps no more than guesswork.

When the trial was done, the jury rejected the psychiatric claims and Chapman was found guilty as charged.

What's The Truth?

The public believes there are special professional tools that can uncover lying, exaggerating, or withholding, but most psychiatrists will admit they have no such tools. It is ironic that the results of a lie detector examination (polygraph) have generally not been accepted by our courts as evidence in trials because of their unreliability, yet psychiatrists regularly testify that their conversations with a criminal defendant have revealed his or her "true" state of mind. If we understand that lie detector examinations are indeed unreliable, it is even harder to justify psychiatry's attempts at lie detection.[15]

What about truth serum? Many lay persons and even some doctors believe that when a drug like sodium amobarbital (Amytal) is injected intravenously in amounts just sufficient to render the person drowsy, he or she will reveal hidden thoughts and will be unable to lie. The results of the interviews are sometimes introduced into a trial. For instance, in a recent case a psychiatrist in Sacramento played for the jury fifteen hours of videotaped interviews of a man injected with Amytal. The taxpayers paid nearly $2,000 not only for the examinations but also for the psychiatrist to sit in the witness chair and watch the tapes with the jury. The psychiatrist justified all this by claiming that Amytal interviews were "a powerful technique for the eliciting of repressed and suppressed memory." In fact, Amytal interviews do not prevent lying, exaggeration, suppression, or manipulation.[16] Rather, they may only create additional problems for a judge or jury. To the extent that Amytal is considered a truth serum, a judge or jury is all the more likely to believe a lie told under Amytal.

If we turn to other techniques, we have no better success. The hypnotic trance, for instance, does not uncover a person's state of mind at the time of a crime. The mysterious and eerie image of the hypnotic process conveyed by films and pulp novels bears no resemblance to the reality.[17] Hypnosis may be a valuable technique for control of pain, anxiety, and even some medical conditions like bleeding disorders; it may be helpful for muscle spasm and in breaking addictions like smoking. But none of this makes hypnosis a tool that can detect lies, bring out "hidden truth," discover multiple personalities, or in any way help a judge or jury, because the hypnotic subject is not asleep and is never under the hypnotist's "control."[18] The subject can lie, fake, or withhold information just as easily as in any other situation. Courtroom psychiatrists who use hypnosis are no more able to help a court get at the truth than are psychiatrists who do not use hypnosis.

Even doctors who have written about these limitations are often willing to go into court and describe their "findings" as though they must be true. Not long ago a psychologist who claimed to have discovered, under hypnosis, the "other" personality in a Marine who raped several preadolescent girls in Hawaii warned other professionals at the same time that "a person is entirely capable of consciously lying under hypnosis."[19] That this is so becomes obvious when several examiners of the same person reach opposite conclusions. During 1977 and 1978 the people of Los Angeles knew that someone in their midst was strangling women and dumping their bodies in the hills surrounding the city. That person became known as the Hillside Strangler. He was finally arrested in Bellingham, Washington, in 1979, after he had killed two more young women; his name was Kenneth Bianchi.

Bianchi entered a plea of legal insanity, and the court ordered the inevitable psychiatric examinations. A total of six experts (five psychiatrists and one psychologist) talked to Bianchi. Psychologist John Watkins, known to have a special interest in the question of multiple personality, claimed to have discovered no fewer than four separate personalities in Bianchi during hypnotic sessions. Most central were the good Ken and the evil Steve. Although it was Kenneth Bianchi who was accused of murder, Watkins said the real culprit was Steve Walker, a vicious alter ego who took control of Bianchi's mind. Steve strangled the victims and then retreated, leaving the good Ken to be blamed for Steve's actions.

This is the stuff of a successful insanity defense. For if a court believed that Ken, the man in the courtroom, was not in control of his behavior, he would be innocent of the murders. Watkins was satisfied that his use of hypnosis allowed him to separate lies from truth: Bianchi was not faking; he was a true multiple personality. Yet an excerpt from one of the interviews using hypnosis clearly indicates that nothing "special" was happening to indicate that Watkins was separating truth from fiction.

WATKINS: Are you the same thing as Ken or are you different in any way? Talk a little louder so I can hear you.

BIANCHI: I'm not him.

WATKINS: You're not him? Who are you? Do you have a name?

BIANCHI: I'm not Ken.

WATKINS: You're not him? O.K. Who are you? Tell me about yourself.

BIANCHI: (No response.)

WATKINS: Do you have a name I can call you by?

BIANCHI: Steve . . . You can call me Steve.

WATKINS: Tell me about yourself, Steve. What do you do?

BIANCHI: I hate him.

WATKINS: You hate him? You mean Ken?

BIANCHI: I hate Ken.

WATKINS: You hate Ken? Why do you hate Ken?

BIANCHI: He tries to be nice . . . I hate a lot of people . . . He tried to make friends.

WATKINS: Who do you hate?

BIANCHI: I hate my mother.

WATKINS: You hate your mother? What has she done to you, Steve?

BIANCHI: She wouldn't let go.
WATKINS: She wouldn't let go. What else do you hate?
BIANCHI: I hate Ken. I hate nice. I hate Ken.
WATKINS: Who's that?
BIANCHI: That's the other person . . . He tries to do good.
WATKINS: Yes, you hate Ken. You hate his mother . . . It's his mother; she's not your mother?
BIANCHI: Well, she is in a way.
WATKINS: What would you like to do about her?
BIANCHI: Disappear.
WATKINS: How do you mean disappear?
BIANCHI: Oh, he likes her being around and I just want her to disappear.
WATKINS: You want her to disappear. Do you get angry?
BIANCHI: Yes.
WATKINS: What do you do when you get angry?
BIANCHI: Anything I can . . . I make him lie . . . I like doing that.
WATKINS: You like to hurt somebody?
BIANCHI: Yeah.
WATKINS: Who do you like to hurt?
BIANCHI: Oh, anybody that's nice to Ken.[20]

By the time each of the doctors had talked with Bianchi and viewed the videotapes of the sessions using hypnosis, the court was ready to poll its experts. The results were two in favor of multiple personality, two against multiple personality, and two undecided.

Supporting Watkins' analysis was Ralph Allison, a psychiatrist who also had a strong interest in the question of multiple personality. Asked how he could be sure "Steve" was real, Allison responded simply, "I met him."[21] A noted expert on hypnosis, Martin Orne, also viewed the videotapes and said, "Bianchi was almost a caricature of a hypnotized person, with eyes closed and head bobbing—a pseudotrance." Psychiatrist Saul Faerstein agreed: Bianchi was faking both the hypnotic state and the multiple personalities. Between these two extremes were two psychiatrists. Donald Lunde decided that Bianchi was not a genuine multiple personality but was a complex man with "at least three faces" to his personality. Charles Moffett did not think Bianchi was faking, at least not consciously, but was not willing to agree to a diagnosis of multiple personality. Rather he declared that Bianchi was a "schizophrenic, undifferentiated type." In describing why he would not go along with the diagnosis of multiple personality, Lunde pointed to what must be regarded as a major flaw in this kind of investigation: Watkins might have invited Bianchi's response. In one session Watkins had said to Bianchi, "If there is some other part of you that wants to talk to me, I'm here to talk to you."

When the doctors were through, the Washington court was many thousands of dollars poorer and could have done as well by flipping coins. That we continue to pay for these opinions says a good deal about the faith we put in psychiatry.[22]

Finally, psychiatrists are sometimes expected to distinguish truths from lies by simply relying on their "clinical experience." But the experienced forensic psychiatrist who has been lied to many times has no way of knowing this and will not learn from experience. If, for example, a murderer falsely tells the psychiatrist that "the voices made me do it," and the psychiatrist accepts this claim, how will the psychiatrist ever learn that he or she was duped? Without corrective feedback, the experienced psychiatrist is just as vulnerable to manipulation as the beginner.

Measuring Current State of Mind

We have now seen that psychiatry is unable to predict future dangerousness and to uncover the truth about a person's past thoughts. Perhaps psychiatrists can describe a person's current capacities more expertly. This is what psychiatrists are asked to do when they testify whether or not a person is fit to stand trial, whether or not a parent is able to raise a child, whether or not a soldier who fails to perform according to expectations is the victim of mental disorder or is merely a shirker. The list of civil, criminal, and administrative procedures that solicit expert psychiatric opinion about current capacity is long. Inevitably the questions come down to this: Is the person mentally disordered? If so, what is the diagnosis and likelihood for recovery? Does the mental disorder render the person incapacitated in some legally relevant manner?

Despite the expectations of many and the assumptions of the law, valid psychiatric evaluation of a person's current mental state is as slippery as a prediction of future behavior or a reconstruction of past motives. Theoretically, the psychiatrist might have a chance to succeed if the profession agreed on what mental disorders are and what to call them. Instead, every ten or fifteen years the American Psychiatric Association publishes a new diagnostic manual because the existing one has proved to be deficient.

The *Diagnostic and Statistical Manual of Mental Disorders* (DSM-1) was first published in 1952. The second edition (DSM-2) was issued in 1968 in a new effort to "stabilize nomenclature in textbooks and professional literature."[23] This might seem to indicate that a stable mode of diagnosis is something to be imposed from above rather than emerge from reliable diagnostic techniques. That conclusion is reinforced by other introductory remarks in the second edition. On schizophrenia, the authors write, "The committee could not establish agreement about what the disorder is; it could only agree on what to call it."[24] A third edition (DSM-3) appeared in 1980.[25] The revision was again the result of a felt need to "stabilize" diagnosis in psychiatry.[26]

Some rather major changes have taken place in psychiatric diagnosis, forcing many to question whether a new diagnostic scheme really solves the problems associated with psychiatric labeling. The most widely publicized change was the removal of homosexuality from the list of officially recognized mental disorders. What particularly struck many observers was the obviously political rather than scientific basis for the change. Under growing pressure from the homosexual community, the trustees of the American Psychiatric Association (APA) declared, by a majority vote in December 1973, homosexuality to be no longer a mental disorder. So much controversy resulted from this that a referendum was called to enable the entire APA membership to vote. Of the total votes cast, 5,854 called for elimination, 3,810 for retention, and 367 abstained.[27] When DSM-3 appeared, homosexuality was once again classified as a mental disorder, but only when the person expressed dissatisfaction with this sexual identity.[28]

Evidence that psychiatric labeling is unreliable and inaccurate has been in existence for a long time, but most of it is buried in professional journals and other publications.[29] One of the most striking articles in this category reports an experiment undertaken in 1973 by David Rosenhan, a Stanford University psychologist. Rosenhan's experiment has done much to alert outsiders that even when psychiatrists agree with each other, they may be wrong.[30]

Rosenhan recruited eight volunteers. They included a psychology graduate student, three psychologists, a pediatrician, a psychiatrist, a painter and a housewife. Each went to the emergency room of a hospital and falsely complained of a single symptom: hearing voices that said "empty," "hollow," and "thud." In every other respect the person acted normally. Every volunteer was admitted to the psychiatric ward. According to plan, after admission each person dropped even the one sham hallucination and simply behaved normally on the ward. Half of the volunteers, following their release weeks later, repeated the experiment at another hospital. Thus, a total of twelve admissions took place.

The results were revealing. Each person was admitted as psychotic; eleven were classified as schizophrenic and one as manic-depressive. It was not a poor reflection on psychiatry that an emergency room psychiatrist, on the basis of one visit, was unable to distinguish between a bona fide psychosis and a fake. Psychiatrists, after all, have plenty to do besides look for researchers with tricks up their sleeves. The disturbing part of Rosenhan's experiment was that after admission to the hospital, although the "patient" showed no abnormal behavior on the ward, the treating psychiatrists were always convinced they were dealing with "a psychotic." The treating psychiatrists were in each case controlled in their evaluations by the diagnosis of the admitting psychiatrist. In all twelve cases, the discharge diagnosis was "schizophrenia, in remission."

As Rosenhan pointed out, this clearly indicated that "once labeled schizophrenic, the pseudopatient was stuck with that label." It also indicated that even if psychiatrists agree with each other, they are hardly free of diagnostic dilemmas. In fact, they may be in even deeper trouble when they start agreeing with each other too regularly. Once a psychiatrist applies a label, correctly or incorrectly, succeeding psychiatrists all too frequently repeat the label.

Psychologist Stephen Morse points out that a major reason for the unreliability of psychiatric labels is that "a diagnosis or label of mental disorder means primarily that a person *behaves* abnormally. Mental disorder does not imply any necessary scientifically proven findings." While medicine measures the body and therefore can collect scientific data, psychiatry's data collection inevitably relies on one person's opinion about another person's behavior. "No test," Morse writes, "will demonstrate the presence or absence of a mental disorder other than the behavior."[31]

Reflections On Psychiatry's Labels

Psychiatric labeling, or diagnosis, will always be more uncertain than diagnosis in medicine. If "diagnosis" in psychiatry is nothing more than one person trying to categorize another, and is not the truly scientific process that occurs in medicine, then a high rate of agreement among psychiatrists may mean the psychiatrists in question are thinking alike rather than identifying and expressing the truth, as Rosenhan's study clearly demonstrates. Because in psychiatry the patient's behavior is *interpreted* by the psychiatrist, whereas in medicine the patient's body may be measured scientifically, there is the possibility that too much consistency in psychiatry resembles a Brave New World more than a genuine breakthrough.

This may sound like a harsh criticism of psychiatry, but it is more closely related to society's wish to give psychiatry the look and feel of science. The greater tragedy is that psychiatry, unlike medicine, does not need this kind of precision. Discrete diagnostic categories are meaningful in medicine because medical diseases exist as discrete and separate entities. Stomach ulcer and stomach cancer may present themselves in a similar manner, but they are concretely different physical processes. Mental disorders are certainly real enough to those suffering emotional pain, and their disordered behaviors are real enough to others. But feelings and behaviors do not come in neat little packages. Mental disorders therefore cannot be "diagnosed" in the same way as medical disorders.

Skepticism about psychiatric "diagnosis" should not imply a nihilistic view of psychotherapy. Emotions, defense mechanisms, personality styles, and maladaptive behaviors do indeed show certain patterns that the experienced therapist may teach to the young trainee. Nonetheless, the ordering of these ideas and the categories and labels used as shorthand do not compare with true medical

diagnoses, which are objectively verifiable labels for physically measurable disorders of the body.

The mode of labeling in psychiatry becomes a serious
concern only when the labels are treated as scientific,
when society invests them with a precision and certainty
they do not have and allows them to influence public policy.
The perpetuation of this error is less an indictment of psychiatry than of society's insistence on using psychiatry in
inappropriate ways. To end this reign of error the state
power associated with psychiatry must be ended.

Lack of scientific tools should be reason enough to
rescind psychiatry's immense legal authority. Yet psychiatry retains its legal hold. Clearly the problem goes deeper
than a mere failure to understand psychiatry's tools. Psychiatry retains its position because the questions our society asks the psychiatrist are scientific in name only. In
reality these questions involve ethical and political dilemmas that groups in society cannot or will not resolve; they
are thus handed over to psychiatry. It is these hidden
agendas that explain psychiatry's immense legal power.

CHAPTER 2

HIDDEN AGENDAS

The abuses that frequently result from giving psychiatry extraordinary legal authority are not primarily the fault of psychiatry but of those of us in society who give psychiatry its power. As a people we use psychiatry to avoid real aims, beliefs, and fears. We hide behind psychiatry's medical cloak of benevolence and science to avoid confronting the true purposes of many of our social policies. In this way it is easier to do certain things without facing why we do them. In exchange, we give psychiatrists immense power and prestige.

What are these hidden aims, beliefs, and fears? First, we deny the truth to ourselves that involuntary psychiatric treatment exists as much for our convenience as for the patient's good. Second, we believe that psychiatry can help reduce the likelihood of unwanted behavior such as violence or suicide and we therefore allow institutions to confine people we are uncomfortable with. Third, we expect psychiatry to resolve apparent technical questions that in truth conceal difficult moral and ethical dilemmas. By taking on these problems, psychiatry absolves society of responsibility for the decision. Fourth, by appealing to the judgment of a professional, we affirm our belief in ourselves as a caring people concerned with individual welfare, even though the decision in question might abuse the civil rights of the person concerned. These illusions have their costs, and the psychiatrist who enjoys the prestige of the profession also bears its burdens.

The Convenience Of Involuntary Treatment

There is no question that benevolence is an element in our belief in involuntary psychiatric treatment. We want to help persons who cannot help themselves. But we have other aims and feelings too. Mentally disordered persons can be a headache and our traditional response has been simply to warehouse large numbers of them. Even today it is often difficult to know when treatment of the patient stops and the convenience of the family or society begins.

No persons are more subject to the mixed feelings associated with involuntary commitment than the family members. Often the family initiates involuntary hospitalization because they experience most vividly the pain, the irrational and unpredictable behavior, the demands, the suffering. They may experience a growing sense of helplessness when their best efforts seem to make no difference. They watch someone who was close to them become distant and alienated. After a while, affection becomes mixed with frustration, embarrassment, and anger. Fatigue sets in, and one's self-protective instincts yearn for relief. Like the mother who has tried everything to soothe a fussing child, family members want to scream, "Enough!"

Outside intervention thus appeals to both love and hate. On the one hand, concern and love cry out for a healer, someone to reverse the process of mental breakdown. On the other hand, frustration and resentment cry out for relief, for rest, for just a little peace. Mental hospitalization, even by force, often seems the best answer. The family finds relief at last but without feeling guilt for having abandoned a member of the family. Others are taking over, professionals who will know what to do— doctors. Psychiatry resolves the family's dilemma by taking control. By forcibly hospitalizing the troubled person the psychiatrist rescues the family, and by calling this treatment society relieves the family of any guilt it might feel for forcibly removing a family member from the home.

This does not mean that loving concern is not also present. In many cases these feelings are very real, but genuine concern is often closely linked with other feelings that are less easily recognized.

If our society should ever consider abolishing involuntary treatment, something that would probably be easier to accomplish than is generally imagined, we would have to pay attention to the dilemmas faced by the family and friends of the mentally disordered. A completely voluntary psychiatry would require alternatives that allow family and friends to separate from the disturbed person, at least for a while, without feeling they have abandoned him or her. Alternatives are possible (see Chapter 9), and would allow us to offer real help to more persons.

Protection of Society

Society looks to the psychiatrist for protection from unwanted or dangerous behavior. We rely on psychiatrists to hospitalize dangerous mental patients, to keep dangerous prisoners from being released too soon, and to hold insane offenders until they are both safe and sane.

While psychiatrists are unable to predict dangerousness, our courts, mental hospitals, and prisons continue to request and use their predictions. Although empowered to write new laws reflecting psychiatry's admitted lack of expertise on dangerousness, legislators show no inclination to do so. Clearly, our reliance on psychiatry to keep us safe is more an irrational hope than a rational conclusion. We have put our faith in today's psychiatrists just as we once put our faith in priests. Neither professional may make us safer, but we *feel* safer. In place of the religious rituals of the past, psychiatrists now perform scientific rituals—"examinations"—to reassure us.

As an example of the function of the ritual of requesting a psychiatric prediction, let us consider the use of psychiatrists in death penalty determinations. In a number of states, death penalty laws require a court to inquire, once a person has been convicted of a crime punishable by death, into the chances that the person will kill again if his or her life is spared. Although none of these laws specifically designates psychiatrists as the ones to advise a judge or jury on its decision, our longstanding reliance on psychiatry has led prosecutors to use professionals in this field to convince a jury to pass the death penalty. One psychiatrist in particular, James Grigson, is well known for his testimony on this issue.[1] Grigson has testified in about sixty cases that the defendant, according to Texas law, "would commit criminal acts of violence that would constitute a continuing threat to society."[2] Perhaps most disturbing is Grigson's awareness that such opinions are not really expert. In an interview he said, "I think the jurors feel a little better when a psychiatrist says it—somebody that's supposed to know more than they know."[3]

While Grigson's role in death penalty trials has been criticized by many, his comment underscores an issue more important than the behavior of one psychiatrist. His statement that "the jurors feel a little better" explains why the psychiatrist is called upon. Not only a jury, but members of society feel safer in following the advice of an "expert." We then feel less guilty about ordering an execution. It is as if the jury, as the representative of the community, were saying, "We have ordered this man be killed, but only after our experts gave their approval."

The recourse to psychiatrists in death penalty hearings is not without challengers. On more than one occasion the practice has been challenged in court by organized psychiatry. On July 6, 1983, the U.S. Supreme Court gave its approval to psychiatric predictions of dangerousness in death penalty hearings.[4] The Court did so even though the American Psychiatric Association (APA) filed an *amicus curiae* brief proclaiming the inability of psychiatrists to predict violent behavior.

Responding to the APA argument that "psychiatrists . . . are incompetent to predict," the Court said, "The suggestion that no psychiatrist's testimony may be presented with respect to a defendant's future dangerousness is somewhat like asking us to disinvent the wheel."[5] The Court later explained what it meant by this: "To accept such argument would call into question other contexts in which predictions of future behavior are constantly made."[6] The Court evidently thought it better to rely on sham examinations than to begin the process of eliminating all psychiatric predictions from courts, mental hospitals, and prisons. The Court may also not have wanted to face the numerous future cases challenging earlier decisions based on psychiatric predictions.

Since psychiatrists make these predictions every day, the Court was saying, our society should continue to use them in death penalty hearings, even if the predictions are worthless.[7] Otherwise the bankruptcy of our society's widespread use of these judgments would become so obvious that dozens of social policies would be suspect. This was the reasoning of our highest court and reflects how strongly our society insists on believing in the powers of psychiatry, whatever the evidence to the contrary. The rituals must go on.

If the highest court in the land lacks the courage to confront the full implications of psychiatry's limitations, it is little wonder that lower courts and legislatures do the same.

But what is easier is often not better. Because of the Court's decision, we must do without a reassessment of laws and social policies based on the false premises of psychiatry's ability to predict future behavior. This means a pervasive unfairness in situations governed by these laws and policies, an unfairness that affects the individual mental patient or prisoner, their families and friends, and society in general.

Freedom from Responsibility

As a society, we ask psychiatrists to make many difficult choices for us. Making choices means taking responsibility for the outcome. If an expert is available to make difficult choices, judges, juries, and administrators are relieved of the burden. Societies, just as much as individuals, want to justify this reliance on experts. Individually or collectively we try to make it appear that we need an expert and that he or she has something special to offer. We exaggerate the expert's skills and minimize our own, thereby disqualifying ourselves from dealing with difficult ethical and moral questions. Let us consider an example.

A seventy-year-old widower, dying of cancer, decided to disinherit his daughter after he learned that she was living with a man out of wedlock. Shortly before his death he altered his will. Having cared for her father during his long illness, the daughter was outraged. She contested his will through the evidence of a psychiatrist, who listened to her story, studied both the new and the old will, and then told a court that her father was "psychotic" at the time of his decision. The charity chosen by her father to receive the money then brought in a psychiatrist who also talked to the daughter and studied the language of the new and old will but concluded that the father was perfectly rational. Neither psychiatrist had talked with the father.

The overt psychiatric questions are, Was the father psychotic? Was his change of heart the product of mental illness? But the deeper, ethical, issues are different: Did the father have a *right* to do whatever he deemed appropriate with his money? Or, did the daughter have an even greater right to claim the inheritance? By relying on psychiatric opinions, the court validates either the father or the daughter, but it does so by focusing on the false issue of psychosis instead of on the ethical and legal issues of right and wrong.

In another example, a sixty-year-old man became despondent. He quit his job and filed for Social Security disability, claiming that he was emotionally unable to work. The examination board, faced with deciding whether the man *could* not work or *would* not work, sent him to a psychiatrist in the hope that the psychiatrist had some expert way of resolving the issue.

Since psychiatrists have no reliable methods to distinguish between those who are mentally disabled and those who are simply fed up with work, recourse to psychiatric opinion only enables society to escape from a difficult ethical dilemma. Are there deserving persons who lack the mental or emotional capacity to care for themselves? Most people agree that there are. But the real issue is, Who are they? How do we identify the deserving and distinguish them from the undeserving? The debate on these questions is so intense that our society has taken the easy way out—we ask a psychiatrist.

Many psychiatrists know they are pawns in this game. In *The Bitter Pill*, Martin Lipp, a physician, tells us about "Warren," a psychiatrist regularly asked to resolve the type of dilemma described above.[8] At a local community mental health center Warren was asked to do a disability evaluation of a forty-two-year-old laborer who claimed to have severe back pain. Orthopedic evaluation showed no evidence of serious disorder, but the man claimed the pain was making him too depressed to work. When he was asked how he would decide whether the man was fed up with twenty-five years of hard labor or was truly "ill" with depression and unable to work, Warren's answer was both frank and revealing. "First, I'm going to go to church and pray for guidance, and then I'll do whatever seems least wrong, and then either way I'll go back to church and confess what I did and pray for forgiveness."[9]

In his frustration, Warren quite understandably tended to blame the patient for the situation. He said,

I have the sense that the disability payment is becoming an end in itself, and people see me only to
give the disability authenticity. Sometimes they
see me solely for the purpose of building a legal
record, so they can say that they had to start seeing a psychiatrist after some traumatic event at
work or a car accident. I see a fair number of patients now who will say, "Be sure and write in my
record that I started having this problem after the
forklift accident." You know exactly what they're
doing. They're building a case for some damn
personal injury lawyer in the workmen's compensation system.[10]

Warren knew he was being "used":

Those people, they don't regard me as a doctor in
any traditional sense. They mostly figure me for
an extension of the court, a bureaucratic function-
ary. They want to see me as briefly as they can,
take care of business, and get out. If anything, they
are more likely to see me as an obstacle to whatever it is they want rather than as help. They've got
to put on as good a performance as possible so that
I'll write something helpful in their record.[11]

Warren recognized that something was wrong, not only
with disability evaluations, but with other evaluations as
well. "Do you know," Warren asked,

how many patients come to see me because they
want anything specifically therapeutic? I'd be surprised if half of them fell into that category. Probably fifty percent are there because they have to
see me for some administrative function I can perform. Like court-ordered competency hearings on
borderline senile old people. I see those by the
dozens. Like exams to see if people are eligible for

aid to the disabled or workmen's compensation. I
bet I see a hundred of those in a year.[12]

What Warren and most other psychiatrists may not
recognize is that in all these examples the fault lies more
with society's habitual dependency on psychiatry than
with the patient. The person seeking a monthly disability
check on the basis of emotional disorder is directed to the
psychiatrist by a caseworker; custom dictates that the
advice of a psychiatrist is needed before anyone can decide
whether or not the person deserves financial support. For
the same reason—our belief that the psychiatrist can offer
expert advice—a criminal defendant claiming he couldn't
help himself is directed by the court to a psychiatrist.

Social custom embodied in our laws and administrative
regulations gives the welfare official, the judge, or the
parole board officer no real choice but to call for psychiatric opinions on difficult questions and to rely on them.
We must all share responsibility for this state of affairs.

Preserving Illusions

As members of a free society, we pride ourselves on our
tradition of supporting the rights of the individual and
restricting the power of the state. Our criminal justice
system—police, courts, jails, and prisons—is supposed to
live by the principles articulated by the Constitution and
by state and local laws. If the criminal justice system does
not always do so, it is because practice often falls short of
theory. Yet we acknowledge that intervention by these
social agencies is intended to benefit society in general,
not the person apprehended.

Through psychiatry, our society cheats on these rules.
How does the mental health system encourage cheating?
It does so by the use of control measures that are labeled
benevolent. Whereas the criminal justice system openly
operates for society's benefit, the mental health system,

specifically, the influence wielded by psychiatry throughout society, claims to operate primarily for the individual's benefit. Courts and legislatures have accepted this rationale of psychiatric controls, and have permitted mental health professionals to follow rules fundamentally different from those governing the criminal justice system. Standards are looser. Factual proof is replaced by psychiatric opinion. Intervention is considered "help" rather than control, and is thus not challenged.

The question is, Why? Why do we use psychiatry in this way? The answer is not easy to confront. A truly free society requires tolerance for people whose behavior leaves us embarrassed, uncomfortable, uncertain—people we may see as fundamentally different from us and therefore not equally entitled to the benefits of our laws. We all want a free society, in the abstract, but in our daily lives it is easy to rely on psychiatric authority to remove from our lives people who are disturbing.

In *The Powers of Psychiatry*, psychiatrist Jonas Robitscher has commented, "Psychiatrists exert power in so many different ways that it is difficult to keep them all in mind."[13] He decided to compile a list of categories but stopped when he had reached fifty-one. In every area where psychiatry is given legal authority to influence official decision making there is a hidden ethical, legal, or political question. Difficult problems are thus avoided temporarily. The following chart outlines the hidden agendas that lie beneath some of the official explanations given for the special powers of psychiatry.

Consequences for the Psychiatrist

More than other doctors, psychiatrists are caught between the wishes of the community and the wishes of their patients. Other doctors have no legal authority to compel patients to accept treatment and are therefore not held responsible for their patients' behavior. Psychiatrists have

Hidden Agendas behind Psychiatric Authority

Legal issue	Official purpose	Hidden ethical, legal, or political agenda
1. Insanity defense	Spare mentally ill offenders from criminal punishment	Reassure ourselves that "mad killers" are not released too soon
2. Psychiatric testimony in death penalty hearings	Offer expert help to the jury on dangerousness	Make it easier to pass a death penalty without feeling guilty
3. Competence for trial	Offer expert help to the judge on the accused's ability to understand charges and assist lawyer	Convenient way to confine without proving guilt; diverting tactic by defense lawyer
4. Involuntary mental hospitalization	Protect mental patients from themselves; protect society from dangerous mental patients	Temporary relief for family and community; convenient control of deviant but noncriminal persons
5. Indeterminate sentencing of criminals	Enhance rehabilitation; release the reformed convict sooner and hold the dangerous convict longer	Control prisoners through uncertainty of release; reassure ourselves that convicts are reformed before release; turn sentencing decisions over to "experts"
6. Juvenile court benevolence	Spare the child the punishing aspects of the adult criminal justice system	Allow more leeway in the control of deviant children, especially members of ethnic minorities
7. Disability evaluation	Expert determination of current capacity for work	Turn over to an "expert" the question whether the person can't work or won't work

legal authority and are expected to use it to protect society from danger and to protect patients from themselves. Psychiatrists may therefore be held partially responsible for the behavior of their patients. This puts enormous pressure on the psychiatrist and leads him or her to rationalize medically what is done in part for self-protection. Let me illustrate these pressures with another example drawn from *The Bitter Pill.*

Lipp talks about "Chris," a psychiatrist whose overwhelming feelings of responsibility for his patients lead Lipp to worry that Chris himself may consider suicide.

> Chris's 7 A.M. patient three days a week is a woman architect who works in a prestigious San Francisco firm . . . Only she and Chris know that she keeps a loaded .30 revolver in her nightstand, not to repel possible intruders, but as the chosen instrument of her suicide. Three times a week as she leaves Chris's office, she says by prior mutual agreement: "I will not kill myself before our next appointment." According to Chris, she says that the only reason she is alive today is because of him; he has kept her from suicide on at least eight separate occasions. She has been seeing him regularly, sometimes as often as seven times a week, for five years.[14]

When Lipp asks Chris how he managed to "save her life," Chris responds, "I love her, and she knows it." Perhaps so, but Chris also knows that society expects him to prevent her suicide. He must do so not only out of concern for her but also out of self-interest.

Chris's patient has him in a hammerlock. He *must* love her or she will kill herself. If she gets angry at him, she can punish and manipulate him by threatening to commit suicide, even acting out the threat. The patient's awareness that society expects psychiatrists to control unacceptable behavior gives the patient the power to manipulate the psychiatrist.

Being held partially responsible for the behavior of patients also pressures the psychiatrist into coercively hospitalizing and treating almost every patient who uses the threat of suicide to manipulate or seems threatening to others. Psychiatrists do not usually enjoy their authority to do so, and are frequently in conflict with their better judgment. A psychiatrist may realize that a concerned but nonetheless firm refusal to take responsibility for controlling the patient is often the very step that would help the patient begin to deal with problems more constructively. But again, the psychiatrist has little choice, because he or she is expected to take over.

Our tendency to hold psychiatrists responsible for their patients' behavior reached the height of absurdity with the claim that since John Hinckley wasn't legally responsible for attempting to assassinate President Reagan— Hinckley being legally insane—someone else was. That someone else was Hinckley's former psychiatrist, John Hopper. Presidential press secretary James Brady, Secret Service agent Timothy McCarthy, and police officer Thomas Delahanty sued Hopper for $14 million, claiming that Hopper should have foreseen Hinckley's assassination attempt and done something to stop it.

On September 16, 1983, Federal district judge John P. Moore dismissed the suit on the grounds that Hopper had no way to anticipate Hinckley's assassination attempt. If this lawsuit had been successful, the rights of thousands of mental patients would have fared even worse than Dr. Hopper's pocketbook. Fearful of such lawsuits, psychiatrists would force patients into mental hospitals even more readily than they do now, and force strong tranquilizers on their patients with even greater frequency. Who could blame a psychiatrist for giving in to this temptation, knowing that a multimillion dollar lawsuit could result any time one of his or her patients does some stupid thing?

If psychiatrists were no longer asked to protect society and individuals from themselves and were confined to practicing their healing art with voluntary patients, psychiatrists would be free to do their best to help their patients without feeling compelled to control their patients out of a sense of self-preservation. This change would allow more persons to receive the help they want and deserve.

Granting legal authority to psychiatrists is poor social policy. The practice of avoiding difficult legal, ethical, and political issues can only lead to injustice and a distortion of our laws and values. Instead of supporting psychiatry as a healing art, we have used it as a tool for shortcuts in solving difficult problems and thereby promoted a system of injustice with consequences that reach far beyond the individuals involved into our courts, mental hospitals, and prisons.

CHAPTER 3

THE INSANITY DEFENSE
Storytelling on the Witness Stand

John Hinckley's acquittal on grounds of insanity made us angry, but it also woke us up. Feelings of outrage and confusion over the insanity plea and courtroom psychiatry in general burst forth. After watching on television Hinckley's attempt to kill President Reagan on March 30, 1981, few people believed that either justice or common sense had prevailed when the jury brought in its verdict. What is more difficult to understand is how and why findings like this one continue to occur. How did psychiatry come to play a crucial role in criminal trials? Why do defense and prosecution psychiatrists often disagree drastically in their expert conclusions? What good, if any, does psychiatry do in our courts? To begin to answer these questions, we must first look at how the insanity defense operates.

Once the defense lawyer decides with the client to enter a plea of not guilty by reason of insanity (known as NGI, sometimes NGRI), the attorney calls in one or more psychiatrists to examine the defendant. Even though the psychiatrists may question the accused weeks or months after the act was committed, they are expected to determine exactly what the defendant was thinking during the moments surrounding the crime. Most particularly, did the accused know what he or she was doing was against the law? If so, was a choice made to commit the crime anyway, or was the behavior beyond the defendant's control? Was he or she driven to it by mental disorder?

Psychiatrists have no tests to reconstruct a past state of mind, but they nonetheless offer an opinion, because they are convinced that their "clinical skills" allow them to expertly determine questions of legal sanity. If they decide the defendant was legally insane at the moment of the crime, the defense lawyer has reason to go forward with an insanity plea. If they decide differently, the defense attorney may decide to start over by hiring another psychiatrist to examine the defendant. A psychiatrist who will reach the desired conclusions can usually be found. Neither judge nor jury learns of the prior psychiatrists, only of those the defense lawyer calls to testify that the defendant was legally insane at the moment of the crime.

If the judge or jury favors the defense psychiatrists' claims of legal insanity over the prosecution psychiatrists' claims of legal sanity, the defendant is found not guilty by reason of insanity and is then sent to a mental institution for an indefinite period of confinement, until at some later date he or she is released as "restored to sanity."

To avoid such an outcome, the prosecutor must try to convince the judge or jury that the defendant indeed understood the criminal nature of the act and also had the capacity to refrain from it but nonetheless chose to commit the crime. Faced with the experts for the defense, the prosecutor also hires one or more psychiatrists, who frequently reach the opposite conclusion: The accused knew right from wrong and had the capacity to refrain from committing the crime.

At the trial, the facts of what actually happened will be presented, but when it comes to whether the person is legally sane and responsible for his behavior, or legally insane and not responsible, the competing claims of the psychiatrists will predominate. Everyone will assume that the psychiatrist is the most qualified to determine such questions. Individual judges or jurors may have some skepticism about psychiatric testimony, but frequently courts are swayed by the very fact that psychiatrists testify as experts and are the only persons allowed to offer opinions on the defendant's innermost thoughts.

With this legal framework as background, let us focus on a particular trial, one that occurred twenty years ago and will provide a useful comparison with today's trials. Readers can supplement my brief comments with the complete story described in Carolyn Anspacher's *The Trial of Dr. De Kaplany.*[1]

The Trial of Dr. De Kaplany

In San Jose, California, an anesthesiologist was in an outrage. Geza de Kaplany had been married to his beautiful wife, Hajna, for only three months when he decided that her lack of sexual enthusiasm was because of an interest in another man. Convinced he was correct in his suspicions, de Kaplany retaliated. From the hospital where he worked he stole three bottles of acid. On the evening of August 28, 1962, he tied his wife to their bed and poured the acid into her eyes, over her face, and onto her groin. As her screams pierced the apartment complex, de Kaplany turned up the radio full volume. Then he went to his neighbors and asked them to forgive him for keeping the radio on so loud. When her screams continued to rise above the noise of the radio, the neighbors called the police. After the police arrived, de Kaplany openly explained, "I wanted to take her beauty away. I wanted to put fear into her as a warning against adultery. Don't worry. She won't die."[2]

According to the testimony of the surgeon who first treated Mrs. de Kaplany:

> Third degree chemical burns covered about 60% of her body; the nipple and surrounding pigmented area of her left breast had been almost completely excised. The cornea of her eyes were so scarred the

pupils were not visible. Most of the external genital area had been burned away.[3]

Thirty-three days later, Hajna de Kaplany died in a San Francisco hospital.

The identity of the killer was no secret. De Kaplany had confessed. Everyone knew too (for neighbors had testified to this at the trial) that he had at the very time his wife was being tortured asked neighbors to forgive the loud music coming from the de Kaplany apartment. Common sense indicated he was trying to conceal his crime by drowning out his wife's screams. De Kaplany must have realized what he was doing was wrong, since he was anxious to cover it up. This knowledge alone was sufficient under then current California law to make de Kaplany legally sane.

Because the evidence was so overwhelming, de Kaplany's attorney entered an insanity plea. His job was now to find psychiatrists and psychologists who would testify that de Kaplany was legally insane. He was able to find the necessary experts, who proceeded to tell the court that de Kaplany had no evil intent when he tortured his wife.

A. Russell Lee tried to convince the jury that the murderer was not even the man sitting in front of them. The real killer was Pierre LaRoche, an "alter ego" who had intermittently lived in the body of de Kaplany since 1945. This was a case of "multiple personality." Lee elaborated:

Geza is courageous, Pierre is a coward. Geza is good, Pierre is bad. Geza is gentle, Pierre is harsh and brutal . . . The motivations of Geza are to help, to rescue, to forgive, to forget, to cure; those of Pierre are to hurt, to abandon, to cause pain, to revenge, to be sadistic and ultimately to commit a sadistic attack.[4]

As far as the crime itself, Lee testified:

> It was really Pierre who went berserk, but it was
> Geza who came to and it was Geza who called the
> ambulance and police. But at the time authorities
> arrived Geza had retreated again, and the calm,
> emotionally fixed man who met them was Pierre.[5]

Interestingly, none of the other professionals hired by the
defense ever claimed they saw or knew anything of this
"alter ego," Pierre LaRoche.

In addition to multiple personality, defense doctors
offered many other explanations in support of the opinion
that de Kaplany had no evil intent and was indeed the innocent victim of mental disorder. Psychologist Robert Zaslow, for example, gave de Kaplany an inkblot test and a
personality questionnaire. At the end of these tests Zaslow
diagnosed de Kaplany as a paranoid schizophrenic, even
though he showed no *outward* signs of being schizophrenic,
that is, of having irrational thoughts (delusions) or hallucinations. The tests, Zaslow was confident, had brought
out the schizophrenic core of de Kaplany's personality.

Zaslow also testified about another psychological test
he had administered, one that showed that de Kaplany had
serious sexual problems. As part of this test, de Kaplany
was asked to define the words *eyes* and *ears*. He had answered that they were "organs of the body." Asked to
define *eggs* and *seeds*, de Kaplany had answered that they
were "something to eat." To Zaslow, these answers were
pathological. *Eyes* and *ears* were not organs of the body,
but *sense* organs of the body, and *eggs* and *seeds* were not
food, but "the beginnings of creation." By these answers
de Kaplany was evidencing a clear wish to deny sexuality.
Here is how Zaslow explained it in his testimony: "This
doctor has a psychosexual disturbance . . . The doctor
has . . . regressed to an oral level of development and therefore is more interested in food, like any one-year-old child,
than in sexual activity."[6] Even if de Kaplany were in fact
more interested in food than in sex, one wonders why the

people of California were paying to hear these opinions in a murder trial.

Zaslow was required to go further. He had to testify as to whether de Kaplany knew, when he was pouring acid on his wife, if his act was against the law. The psychologist testified, "[De Kaplany] did not understand the social significance of what he did or that he would be punished or how other people would feel about it. In the test material he showed confusion between right and wrong."[7] Finally, while Zaslow concentrated on eggs and seeds, he found no evidence of de Kaplany's supposed dual personality. If Lee had found the alter ego Pierre LaRoche so readily accessible, why had Zaslow found no evidence of him at all?

Psychiatrist Lindsay C. Beaton took the witness stand next, bringing to the jury yet another set of psychiatric notions concerning the killer. Beaton said that de Kaplany was destined from early childhood to commit the act. "There are certain bright threads running through the fabric of his life, which point to the unavoidable commission of what he finally did."[8] This would imply, of course, that de Kaplany was not responsible for his behavior, since everything he did was "unavoidable." Beaton went on to testify: "I don't think that at the deep levels of his personality the doctor was really killing his wife."[9]

Who, then, was he killing? His mother, of course. After deciding that de Kaplany was a "latent homosexual" who was in conflict with his mother, Beaton claimed, "This unconscious feeling, combined with the problem about his mother, swept this particular psychotic individual into a symptom which in his case was a criminal act—murder."[10]

When the defense psychiatrists were through, the prosecution called three psychiatrists of its own. Each of these doctors—also supposed experts—came to conclusions diametrically opposed to those of the defense psychiatrists. According to the three prosecution psychiatrists, de Kaplany was perfectly sane; he had indeed been capable of knowing right from wrong at the moment of his crime.

The conflicting psychiatric testimony added up to twelve volumes, 250,000 words, and many thousands of dollars of the taxpayers' money. None of this expense was necessary. The jury only had to look at the facts of the case before them: First, de Kaplany had confessed to the torture, with the words "I wanted to take her beauty away." Second, de Kaplany's neighbors testified that he had asked them to overlook the loud radio music, indicating he knew very well what he was doing: He was consciously trying to drown out his wife's screams.

The jury found de Kaplany guilty of first-degree murder, showing that juries do not always accept the claims of defense psychiatrists. De Kaplany spent ten years in prison and was then paroled.

This hardly means that an injustice did not take place. Even when the psychiatric claims of "dual personality" or speculations about "eggs and seeds" failed to convince a judge or jury, the taxpayers' pocketbook was still victimized. Regardless of the verdict, we paid for testimony that was not required, because the plain facts of the defendant's behavior were more than sufficient to allow a fair verdict to be reached.

The confusion and needless expense of the insanity defense have not lessened in the twenty years since de Kaplany's trial. If anything, things are worse. The role of psychiatry in criminal trials has expanded. Unlike twenty years ago, most states now ask the psychiatrist not only whether the accused knew right from wrong but also whether he had the "substantial capacity to conform his conduct to the requirements of the law." The psychiatrist comments, in other words, on whether the person acted with free will. For centuries wise men and philosophers have been debating the question of free will, so it should hardly be surprising to find that psychiatrists have not discovered the answer.

The trial of John Hinckley illustrates that in some jurisdictions, such as the federal courts and a few states, the confusion arising from this question runs even deeper. The prosecution had to prove beyond a reasonable doubt that Hinckley acted with free will, whereas in most states the defendant is presumed to be legally responsible until proven legally insane. Free will, or the capacity to control one's behavior, can never be proven scientifically, because it is a metaphysical concept rather than a scientific fact. Free will is an *idea*, not a tangible substance to be measured or "examined." To ask a prosecutor to prove that a crime was committed with free will is to ask the impossible. When this question becomes the focus of psychiatric testimony, a fiasco is all too likely.

What's Going Wrong?

Trials like John Hinckley's have at least raised public consciousness about courtroom psychiatry. Many people are angry about psychiatric testimony and feel basic reform is needed, but are unsure what is required. The leaders of forensic (legal) psychiatry agree that problems abound, but they certainly do not acknowledge that these problems stem from a lack of true scientific tools available to the psychiatrist. They argue instead that courtroom psychiatrists need *better training* in the skills that forensic psychiatry already has. Seymour Pollack, a leader in forensic psychiatry, put it this way in testimony before a California legislative committee investigating "the role of psychiatry in determining criminal responsibility."

> I would like to stress how necessary it is for there to be support by the state for training and educational programs in this field . . . because at the present time these skills are not taught nor are they developed by the average psychiatrist or psychologist . . . And that's one of the reasons we have such terrible results.[11]

If Pollack is correct, trials featuring the most highly qualified psychiatrists, rather than the average psychiatrist, should avoid "such terrible results." Yet the testimony of the best psychiatrists in forensic psychiatry does not differ from that of their less famous colleagues. The trial of Robert Kennedy's killer, Sirhan Sirhan, can serve as an example.

With no real question that Sirhan was the killer, a mental defense was entered on his behalf. His lawyers argued that when he killed Kennedy and wounded several others, on June 4, 1968, Sirhan was suffering from a mental disorder that prevented him from being capable of deliberately planning a murder. The featured witness for the defense was Bernard Diamond, professor of law and criminology at the University of California's prestigious Boalt Hall of Law, professor of psychiatry at the University of California Medical School in San Francisco, and one of the world's foremost forensic psychiatrists.

Diamond spared no effort. In an interview after the trial, he estimated that he had "worked with him [Sirhan] twenty to twenty-five hours."[12] In addition to talking with Sirhan, Diamond tried hypnosis and liquor in hopes of prying loose Sirhan's intent when he shot Kennedy. The results of these investigations led Diamond to conclude that Sirhan had trained himself to go into a hypnotic trance with the help of mirrors and candles. And these trances supposedly explained Sirhan's notebooks in which he had written "R.F.K. must die" and "Robert F. Kennedy must be assassinated before June 5, 1968."

How did the alleged trances relate to these death threats? The threats, Diamond asserted, came from Sirhan's *unconscious* mind, not his conscious mind. And Sirhan should not be held responsible for behavior that sprang directly from the unconscious mind. Diamond explained it this way:

> After going into a trance thinking of love and peace, he would emerge to find his notebook filled with incoherent threats of violence and assassina-

tion. He would have no recollection of having written anything but knew that it was his handwriting . . . In his unconscious mind there existed a plan for the fulfillment of his sick, paranoid hatred of Kennedy and all who might want to help the Jews. In his conscious mind there was no awareness of such a plan or that he, Sirhan, was to be the instrument of assassination.[13]

Yet despite Sirhan's unconscious impulses, Diamond claimed, Kennedy's death was still more a matter of terrible coincidence than a deliberate political assassination.

Sirhan ended up half-drunk on gin—Tom Collinses— at the hotel late on the night of June 4, when Kennedy won the primary. By the least likely accident of all he blundered into an alcove lined with mirrors and wall lights, which trapped him into his dissociated state. A few more blunders took him by a circuitous route into that pantry shortly before Kennedy happened to come through.[14]

This was, supposedly, courtroom psychiatry at its "best." The great amount of time spent examining Sirhan and Diamond's impeccable credentials were just what the leaders of psychiatry said were necessary in every case.

Why *do* courtroom psychiatrists so frequently offer such farfetched testimony? Because psychiatrists do not have the tools to find out what an accused person was thinking at the time of the crime. The psychiatrist can and does talk to the defendant and sometimes reads information gathered by police. But when it comes to deciding whether at the moment of the crime the accused knew right from wrong, the psychiatrist can do this no better than anyone else. There are no tests to determine the past state of mind of another human being, and there is no expert way of distinguishing truth from lies. Psychologist William Winslade, in *The Insanity Plea*, put it this way:

> We ask the expert in this area, a psychiatrist, to rescue us from this troublesome area of judging our fellow citizens and their actions. And the psychiatrist has responded to this impossible request. He has obligingly provided us with his own confusion—no different from our own—but he presents it in an appealingly expert way, with special language and special tests to validate his special knowledge. Unfortunately, it takes more than tests and fancy language to create special, expert knowledge.[15]

After questioning lawyers, judges, and jurors, I have concluded that in many trials both judge and jury are skeptical of the psychiatric opinions they hear. But jurors go home after the trial and are not in a position to change the laws that invite the psychiatrist into the courtroom. Judges are also unlikely to voice their skepticism except in the privacy of their chambers. They certainly may not try to influence jurors' opinions of each testifying psychiatrist. Those who *are* in a position to do something about the insanity defense—state and federal legislators—have indeed grappled with these problems from time to time, as have innumerable blue-ribbon commissions. But previous reforms have failed to solve the problems because lawmakers and reformers have been unwilling to consider the possibility that the problem is not *how* psychiatric testimony enters into a trial but that it enters at all. No legislature has yet given serious consideration to a ban on psychiatric testimony, perhaps because legislators have not yet recognized that there is a better way to determine criminal intent—attention to the defendant's behavior immediately prior to, during, and immediately after the crime.

Instead of considering this alternative, legislators and reformers have tried, again and again, to devise a new definition of legal insanity in the hope that this would somehow solve the problem of the insanity defense.

Defining Insanity

The term *insanity* is used in the courtroom to mean something very different from what it has meant over the years, both medically and popularly. Medically, *insanity* used to refer to those symptoms that we now label *psychotic* or *schizophrenic*, such as delusions (irrational thoughts) or hallucinations. Today *insanity* is no longer a medical term. But it is still a legal term.

In about half the states *insanity* is legally defined as the inability to understand the wrongful or criminal nature of the act committed.[16] This use of the term emerged in 1843, when Daniel M'Naughten attempted to kill British prime minister Robert Peel. He did not succeed, but killed Peel's secretary instead. M'Naughten's attorney successfully argued that at the time of the shooting M'Naughten had a mental disorder that prevented him from understanding that his actions were wrong.[17] Although this was by no means the first time an "insanity" defense had been used in England, the trial was unusual for *the role of expert testimony* in determining the state of mind of the accused.[18] M'Naughten's lawyer heavily relied on the book *A Treatise on the Medical Jurisprudence of Insanity*, in which the American physician Isaac Ray argued that doctors should play a key role in any trial in which legal insanity was an issue.[19] Before this time, the testimony of eyewitnesses or acquaintances was the principal basis upon which a judge or jury rendered a verdict.

Today the insanity defense relies almost exclusively on the testimony of psychiatrists. When they offer opinions about whether or not an accused person knew right from wrong at the time of the crime, this is called the M'Naughten test, and in many states this "right-wrong" test still defines legal insanity. For many years psychiatrists expressed discomfort with this test, saying that it failed to take account of unconscious and irresistible impulses. What they wanted was a new test, and they got it in 1954 when a federal court expanded the definition of legal insanity.

The "Product" Test

Psychiatrists pointed out that the "right-wrong" test for insanity was hopelessly out of date because the psychoanalytic revolution had deepened our understanding of how the mind works. Freud had demonstrated that behavior was not merely the result of conscious decisions based on rational thinking. The unconscious mind was a powerful, if hidden, influence on behavior. Furthermore, it was the ability to understand how the unconscious workings of the mind controlled a person's behavior, especially deviant behavior, that set the psychiatrist apart from everyone else. It was here that the psychiatrist could make a real contribution to an insanity trial. If a psychiatrist's talents were wasted on merely determining whether a person knew right from wrong, both science and justice would suffer. A person might know right from wrong but be unable, because of mental disorder, to control his or her specific acts.

A well-known authority described the general discontent psychiatrists felt with the M'Naughten "right-wrong" test of insanity.

> We have reached a place where there is a consensus that the M'Naughten test of responsibility in the defense of insanity is no longer useful. The Royal Commission on Capital Punishment conceded that "the test of responsibility laid down by the M'Naughten rule is so defective that the law on the subject ought to be changed." In this country [U.S.] the Criminal Law Advisory Committee of the American Law Institute has likewise viewed the M'Naughten rule. To these views now expressed from the side of the law may be added an almost unanimous expression of dissatisfaction on the part of the profession of psychiatry.[20]

Psychiatry was quite capable of bringing "modern thinking" into the insanity trial if only the legal definition of insanity were modernized. Let the psychiatrist inform the court not only whether the defendant knew the act was wrong but also whether the defendant was capable of restraint; then the confusion would end.

In 1954 this reasoning culminated in the *Durham* rule, written by the highly respected federal appeals court judge David Bazelon.[21] It said, "An accused is not criminally responsible if his unlawful act was *the product* of mental disease or mental defect" (emphasis added). A person could, in other words, know his behavior was wrong yet still be driven to it by mental disorder.

This ruling was what the psychiatrists had long been waiting for. What made them particularly happy was the key phrase "the product of mental disease." Far from restricting the psychiatrists, as the M'Naughten test had done, this phrase allowed them much greater leeway to testify about unconscious forces acting at the time of the crime. These hidden forces were, of course, precisely why psychiatrists were needed in trials on legal insanity. Not surprisingly, the response from the psychiatric community was enthusiastic. Law professor Alexander Brooks explains,

> Articles were written in both psychiatric and legal journals by psychiatrists unstintingly praising the new test as a revelation of enlightenment . . . Karl Menninger, for instance, acclaimed the *Durham* rule as "more revolutionary in its total effect than the Supreme Court decision regarding segregation." Judge Bazelon was awarded a certificate of commendation by the American Psychiatric Association.[22]

Despite this early enthusiasm, the *Durham* rule was not widely accepted by the courts. Other judges quickly realized that instead of bringing psychiatric testimony under control, *Durham* only allowed it to get out of hand. If *all* behavior was, as Freud taught, the result of predetermined unconscious forces, it was easy for any crime to be interpreted as the result of hidden mental forces and thus the "product" of mental disorder. The result of *Durham* was a huge increase in findings of legal insanity in the District of Columbia, something no one really desired.

Irresistible Impulse Test

Lawyers and leading forensic psychiatrists accepted the unworkability of the *Durham* rule and tried to find another definition of legal insanity. In 1962 the American Law Institute (ALI) came up with this:

> A person is not responsible for criminal conduct if at the time of such conduct as a result of mental disease or defect, he lacked substantial capacity either to appreciate the criminality (wrongfulness) of his conduct or to conform his conduct to the requirements of law.[23]

This definition, commonly called the ALI test, was supposed to avoid the ambiguities of the *Durham* rule. Psychiatrists would now determine whether the defendant either was incapable of knowing right from wrong, *or could not help himself* and was compelled to commit the crime because of mental illness. This was the "irresistible impulse" test, in truth no different from the "product of mental disease" test of *Durham*. In 1972 the Supreme Court gave the new definition of legal insanity its stamp of approval, setting the stage for its eventual adoption by the states.[24]

Have these changes in the legal definition of insanity made any real difference in what happens when psychiatrists are called to testify? By general agreement, they have not. Insanity trials still come down to a battle between expert opinions that seem more the product of speculation than science. A recent case in a state that accepts the ALI test for legal insanity will illustrate this point.[25]

A well-established psychiatrist testified that when the accused, "Tony," stabbed and killed his wife, he was temporarily insane. The wife had threatened to leave Tony many times, and he had threatened to kill her rather than let her go. These threats had worked in the past, but this time she was determined to leave. As she packed her things, he stabbed her repeatedly until she died. After a neighbor alerted the police, Tony confessed to the crime in a coherent and rational manner. He did not appear delusional or out of touch with reality in any way, either to the police or to his coworkers, friends, and neighbors.

The psychiatrist testifying for the defense nevertheless explained that the threatened loss of his wife caused Tony to experience a temporary loss of contact with reality. The psychiatrist called this a dissociative reaction. While in this state Tony killed his wife; after the deed he immediately returned to reality.

When he was later questioned on cross-examination, the psychiatrist made the claim that Tony remained sane until one second before he made the first stab wound. Then, he remained insane until one second after he made the last stab wound. Then he regained his sanity and has been lucid ever since.

For most people, common sense alone dictates that we reject such fanciful speculations. Yet the fact remains that incredible psychiatric testimony of this sort is not at all unusual, and in this case Tony was pronounced legally insane by the judge. Once again, William Winslade, in *The Insanity Plea*, explains in part why this testimony occurs:

> When psychiatrists are not allowed to testify about whether or not the defendant actually understood what he was doing, they begin to testify about whether he had the capacity to understand what he was doing. If that is forbidden, they start testifying about whether he had the capacity to intend harm. The focus of their testimony changes slightly, but the testimony is no more precise, no less misleading, and no more likely to avoid injustice.[26]

What's happening? Why haven't trials of legal insanity become rational affairs, despite the constant redefinition of legal insanity? The reform proposals of legal experts and legislators have been too superficial. These proposals have taken the need for psychiatric testimony as a given, something beyond question. The problem is not so much the definition of legal insanity as the *method* by which the court decides the issue. As long as psychiatric reconstructions are allowed, the confusion will continue regardless of which definitions of legal insanity are adopted.

The Hidden Purpose of the Insanity Defense

Despite our difficulties with the insanity defense, it continues, for it serves an unspoken function. The insanity defense exists not to excuse the mentally disordered offender from criminal responsibility, as legal theory teaches, but to make all of us feel safer. The irrational offender frightens us more than the rational offender; we have therefore made provisions whereby certain offenders, labeled legally insane, are sent to a mental institution rather than to a prison. We assume that psychiatrists at the mental hospital will treat the person until he is "sane" once more and no longer dangerous. In essence, we rely on the insanity defense not because we wish to excuse some offenders, but because we believe it offers us, through the role of the psychiatrists, better protection from future crimes than an ordinary prison sentence offers.

This conclusion is admittedly a speculation, but it is the result of listening to people's reactions when I recommend that all criminal offenders, even those suffering from mental disorders, be given determinate (fixed) rather than indeterminate sentences. I recommend that offenders be released at the expiration of this definite sentence, with no opportunity for society to extend confinement on the basis of alleged dangerousness. It is this recommendation, rather than my call for a ban on psychiatric testimony, that many people find frightening. They respond, "What if the offender is still dangerous?" I then remind them that neither psychiatrists nor anyone else can tell who is still dangerous, so the sentence should be based on what the offender *has done*, not on what he *might do*.

At this point a crucial thing happens. Despite my arguments about the lack of any way to predict dangerousness, listeners *nonetheless want psychiatric evaluations to continue*. In one way or another they say, "Well, there must be *some* way." Or, "Probably no one can do it any better than the psychiatrists." Or, "We can't simply release insane killers just because a definite sentence has expired."

Although we have to some extent succumbed to emotion in the case of ordinary (legally sane) offenders, and adopted indeterminate sentences for them too, the fear of adopting a policy of definite release is far greater in the case of legally insane offenders. This special fear of the "mad killer" prompts us to retain the insanity defense, a device that seems to guarantee us protection from the irrational criminal.

We explain the insanity defense to each other by saying that legally insane criminals are being protected from criminal punishment. Excused from criminal blame, they are to be treated, not punished. But closer reflection quickly reveals that confinement in a mental institution is just as much a punishment as is confinement in a prison. And it is quite possible for an offender found legally insane to be confined *longer* in a mental institution than a person found guilty of the same crime and confined in a prison.

How and why has this happened? How has it come about that a person found "not guilty" may be punished as much as or more than one found "guilty"? The answer lies in the history of criminal punishment. When the insanity defense originated hundreds of years ago, it had the effect of saving the legally insane offender from execution, for at that time the punishment for serious crime was death.[27] To protect public safety, the legally insane person was not released but was incarcerated in an asylum for life. By today's standards this is harsh treatment, but the practice did keep some from going to their deaths. In this sense, then, a finding of insanity was an act of clemency that excused the legally insane offender from the most severe and traditional form of punishment—death.

Today the death penalty is seldom used; it has been replaced by a prison sentence. Thus, when we put legally insane offenders into a mental institution, they are receiving essentially the same *punishment* as those found legally sane—confinement. There are differences: Physical conditions in prisons are generally harsher, but in other ways the mental institution may be more punishing than prison. Forced administration of mind-altering drugs, for example, is more prevalent in mental hospitals than in prisons. Most important, both to the offender and to society, is the question of *how long* the confinement lasts. To a greater degree than is the case for legally sane prison inmates, the legally insane hospital inmate is at the mercy of psychiatric evaluations. Ironically, society is also at the mercy of the evaluations.

Safety Through Psychiatry

To win release from the mental hospital, a legally insane offender must go through a second sanity trial. Now it is the state's attorney who uses psychiatric testimony to argue that the person is very sick. The inmate is, in fact, dangerous and must not be released. The defense lawyer counters with psychiatrists who say the person is restored to sanity and is no longer dangerous.

The outcomes of these trials are varied. By relying on psychiatric pronouncements on dangerousness, instead of passing sentences based on the seriousness of the crime committed, courts may release a murderer after just a few months or perhaps a year or two.[28] Meanwhile, the same courts may confine for much longer terms other offenders whose crimes did not involve death or bodily injury. Our reliance on psychiatry is thus hardly making us safer. Let us consider the record in New York state, for example. Murderers found legally insane between 1965 and 1976 were released, on the average, in less than eighteen months. One murderer spent just *one day* in the hospital, whereas another person whose crime was possession of a weapon was held nearly two and a half years.[29] In New Jersey, murderers found insane were released in just two years, on the average.[30]

The data from New York are revealing in other respects as well. Besides showing a "dramatic increase in the number of insanity acquittals since 1971," they also indicate that whites are more likely to benefit from psychiatric testimony than are blacks. While whites make up only 30 percent of the state's prison population, they constitute 60 percent of those found not guilty by reason of insanity.[31] These data are important, but they do not tell the whole story. They speak of *averages*, whereas both criminals and their victims are *individuals*. If one murderer is released after one year, and another after nine years, the average is five years. One person is locked up nine times longer, but this fact is completely lost in the averaged figure.

The root cause of this injustice is the fact that psychiatric speculations on "dangerousness" are the determining factor in how long the person is held. This practice leads to situations that violate common decency and justice.

An excellent example is Thomas Vanda, a man who profited from the insanity defense and may one day write a book about it. He has already written a letter on the subject, and demonstrated considerable knowledge of its subtleties. In 1971, Vanda murdered a fifteen-year-old girl, but was found not guilty by reason of insanity and sent to a mental institution. Released only nine months later, he was subsequently accused of another murder, the fatal stabbing of twenty-five-year-old Marguerite Bowers. While in custody, he sent a letter to a friend who was also in jail on charges of murder. Vanda entitled his letter "How to beat a murder rap by insanity."[32]

1. Get a psychiatric examination such as: "inkblot test" and come up with some way out things to say as to what those inkblots look like to you.
2. Tell doctors you are hearing voices and what those voices were saying to you, such as, say those voices told you to do your crime.
3. Make it look convincing. Do not give any indication that you are faking.
4. Act crazy in front of the staff.

Vanda even offered his friend some examples of how to carry it off.

1. Say the inkblots look like two men having sex with each other.
2. Tell doctors the voices say to break out in hysterical laughter. Then break out in hysterical laughter.
3. Masturbate in front of the staff members.

Vanda was pleading legal insanity for the second offense and Edward Keller, chief of Chicago's Cook County Psychiatric Institute, had already concluded that Vanda was legally insane. When Vanda's letter was discovered, Keller was asked if this would change his opinion. The letter, the doctor responded, was no cause for altering his earlier finding.[33]

Edmund Kemper provides another example of how little we can expect psychiatrists to protect us from the violent criminal. As an adolescent, Kemper had killed both his grandparents. Sent to an institution for a few years, he was released but required to return for periodic examinations. His last examination, which certified him as "safe," was done while he was in the midst of committing an as yet undiscovered string of eight murders.[34]

Events that took place on Thanksgiving Day 1976 offer yet another example. On that day, a white New York police officer, Robert Torsney, shot and killed black fifteen-year-old Randolph Evans. Evans was not armed. Charged with murder, Torsney entered a plea of not guilty by reason of insanity, claiming that at the moment of the crime he blacked out. Defense psychiatrists then testified that Torsney had been suddenly overtaken by an epileptic seizure. They said that epilepsy of the psychomotor type predisposes one to violence, a claim with no scientific basis.[35] Torsney, moreover, had no previous history of epilepsy. Nevertheless, the all-white jury accepted the story. Found not guilty by reason of insanity on November 26, 1976, Torsney was sent to the Creedmoor Psychiatric Center in Queens. After one year, he was allowed to spend most of his nights and weekends at his nearby home. By July 1978, after eighteen months, he was released. The doctors at Creedmoor never found any evidence of epilepsy, either on the night Torsney killed Randolph Evans or at any other time. They declared that Torsney was no longer dangerous. According to law, he therefore had to be released.[36]

The case of Clara Gordon illustrates just how far justice may be perverted by our current policies. She confessed to killing Sharon Reid by stabbing her sixteen times. Two out of three psychiatrists testified that Gordon was insane at the time of the crime, and Judge Kenneth Wendt of the Circuit Court of Cook County found her not guilty by reason of insanity. Sent to Chicago's Reed Mental Health Center, Gordon was observed by a psychiatrist, who decided she was no longer dangerous. After only one week of confinement, she was released.[37]

We have no national statistics on how often these things happen, but the New York and New Jersey studies indicate that murderers found insane may be released from a mental institution in a year or two—a much shorter time than they would have spent in prison. Because psychiatry has officially proclaimed its inability to predict dangerousness, it is a cruel hoax on society to release murderers on the word of a psychiatrist. A confinement of a year or two, moreover, hardly seems adequate punishment for a person who has brought to an end the life of another. It is equally unfair when nonviolent offenders found legally insane are locked up until a psychiatrist declares them safe. These persons may remain locked up for years. In some states, the courts have addressed themselves to this problem, but the solutions have been less than adequate. The California Supreme Court, for example, ruled in the case of *In re Moye*, "The duration of institutional confinement of such persons cannot exceed the maximum term for the underlying offense."[38] So far so good, but then the court added that the inmate must be released "unless the people or other committing authority establish grounds for an extended commitment." How would such grounds be established? Through the use of psychiatric examinations and testimony on dangerousness. This means that even if other states follow California's lead and make it more difficult on paper to confine the legally insane longer in mental hospitals than the legally sane in prisons, the injustice will still continue. And despite psychiatry's formal acknowledgment that dangerousness is not a subject within its expertise, there is no shortage of psychiatrists willing to render opinions on this question in court. It is thus not unusual for a legally insane criminal to be kept longer in an asylum than a legally sane criminal in a prison.

Let us consider the case of an inmate I'll call Fred. In 1973 he was found not guilty by reason of insanity after firing a weapon into an inhabited dwelling. No one was hurt. He was sent to Atascadero State Hospital in California. On several occasions during the next five years, Fred attempted to gain release by proving to a court that he had regained his legal sanity—that is, he was no longer dangerous. Unsuccessful each time, he finally applied for release when he had served the maximum time he could have been given if found guilty and sane. Under the recent *Moye* decision, Fred should have been released "unless the people or other committing authority establish grounds for an extended commitment."

More than ten years after his confinement began, Fred is still locked up. I have on two occasions interviewed him and then testified that the predictions of institutional psychiatrists, claiming Fred was still dangerous, were not valid, scientific predictions. Every year or two, when Fred tries again, the jury turns him down. The reason? Fred is chronically psychotic. He is preoccupied with various color combinations and geometric patterns and is convinced these are being used, via the television, to control his mind.

Persons like Fred are typical of legally insane offenders who are likely to be incarcerated longer than offenders found guilty and sane and sent to prison. The trial for release focuses supposedly on dangerousness, but it is simply unheard of for hospital psychiatrists to recommend release of a convict still psychotic. When it is remembered that persons in Fred's condition are not more likely to be dangerous than rational offenders, the injustice becomes clear.[39]

By using the insanity defense to pursue "safety through psychiatry," we arrive at the following: Chicago's insanity expert and murderer, Thomas Vanda, was rational and coherent, so much so that he easily fooled psychiatrists into considering him "restored to sanity" and ready for release only nine months after his first murder. Had he been irrational (psychotic) he could not have convinced the psychiatrists. He then killed again. Fred, on the other hand, has never killed anyone. His crime resulted in no physical harm. But because he *is* irrational, he has little chance to convince psychiatrists he is a safe bet for release. Safety through psychiatry means our society is just as likely to release a vicious and clever, but nonpsychotic, killer as we are to confine indefinitely a relatively harmless, but psychotic person.

Psychiatry Responds

The Hinckley verdict was an embarrassment to psychiatry, for the kind of courtroom speculations that usually go unnoticed were brought before the entire nation. Forced to save face, the American Psychiatric Association (APA) decided to issue a special report on the insanity defense.[40] A brief look at its recommendations will help us decide whether the leaders of psychiatry can get us out of our current mess, or whether we should look elsewhere for truly progressive reform.

The APA's first recommendation is that we return to the M'Naughten "right-wrong" test for legal insanity, and abandon the attempt to decide if a defendant had the "capacity to conform" his or her behavior:

> Many psychiatrists . . . believe that psychiatric information relevant to determining whether a defendant understood the nature of the act, and whether he appreciated its wrongfulness, is more reliable and has a stronger scientific basis than . . . psychiatric information relevant to whether a defendant was able to control his behavior. The line between an irresistible impulse and an impulse not resisted is probably no sharper than that between twilight and dusk.[41]

The leaders of psychiatry are thus saying that their recommendation *during the past one hundred years*, right up to the Hinckley trial, was misguided, even though it was the lobbying of psychiatrists that convinced lawmakers and judges to abandon the M'Naughten "right-wrong" test in favor of the "irresistible impulse" test. "Get rid of M'Naughten," psychiatry said, "and the insanity defense will work fine." Now psychiatry says, "Give us back M'Naughten and the insanity defense will work fine." What official psychiatry will not say, of course, is that *any* test that relies on psychiatric testimony about *anything* will continue to produce the same courtroom circus.

The other major recommendation of the APA report concerns what should happen to the person found legally insane. The APA suggests conditional release, or parole, when there is "a coherent and well structured plan of supervision, management, and treatment" available, one that is "highly likely to guarantee public safety" and that includes "a procedure to reconfine the insanity acquittee who fails to meet the expectations of the plan."[42] This plan, already adopted in Oregon and highly touted in the media, would offer us the worst of both worlds. That is, release would still be based on unreliable predictions of dangerousness, and once released these persons would be subjected to the tyranny of unchecked psychiatric power. They would be forced to take powerful tranquilizing drugs indefinitely and to face reconfinement whenever they were "uncooperative," or whenever they would not "accept treatment." Society, moreover, would receive violent offenders back into its midst because a "treatment plan" was felt to justify release, not because a sentence fitting the crime had been completed. Once again the advice of psychiatry will lead us down the path of injustice and confusion. Something very different is clearly needed.

Ending the Insanity Defense

Experts from psychiatry and law have failed to adequately define the relationship between these two professions because they fail to acknowledge the hypocrisies of the insanity defense. In summary, these hypocrisies are

1. The justification for the insanity defense—that legally insane persons should neither be blamed nor punished: These persons *are* punished, by incarceration in a mental institution.

2. The mode of determining legal insanity—through psychiatric testimony: The psychiatrist has no special way of telling what a person was thinking, or of evaluating capacity, when that person committed a crime.

3. The reliance on psychiatric predictions to protect society: Indefinite psychiatric confinement is unjust, both to society when the confinement is too short for the crime committed, and to the offender when the confinement is too long for the crime; furthermore, confinement based on psychiatric guesswork about dangerousness neither protects society nor allows real therapy for criminals who happen to have psychological problems.

Abolition of the insanity defense would *not* mean that courtroom decisions on criminal intent *(mens rea)* would be eliminated from the criminal law, as is often assumed by even highly sophisticated legal scholars. On the contrary, courts of law will inevitably need to decide the intent behind many kinds of crime. Negligent homicide secondary to drunk driving, for example, is hardly the same crime as premeditated murder, even though both are major crimes and call for serious punishment. But in determining what, if any, criminal intent was present, and in deciding punishment, our judges and juries need no help from psychiatrists.

How should intent be determined? A decision on intent should be based on the factual evidence surrounding the crime. For the evidence surrounding a crime is really no different from the evidence surrounding our daily lives. And each day we make many inferences about a person's mental intent. We do so by judging what he does and how he does it, what he says and how he says it. If, for example, I am standing in the checkout line at the supermarket and I feel myself pushed from the side, I will turn and by virtue of what I see and hear I will decide the intent of the person who has bumped me. If the person apologizes and motions me to go ahead, I conclude that it was an accident. If the person insists that he or she was ahead of me, or simply looks straight ahead and inches forward, I conclude something very different. I may be wrong in my conclusion, or someone else standing in line may have seen and heard the same things and put the information together differently. But neither of us is an "expert," even if one of us happens to be a psychiatrist.

We make judgments like this every day outside the courtroom, and there is no reason that a judge or jury cannot do the same inside the courtroom. Although the stakes are much higher in court, the fact remains that we have no better way to determine mental intent other than by simply examining the factual evidence concerning what the accused person did and how he or she did it. The judge and jury are already given responsibility to be the "trier of fact," that is, to make the final decisions. Our current laws, thus, say that expert testimony is not the final word in deciding the issue of mental intent. The judge or jury gives expert testimony a little weight or a lot, depending on how credible the testimony seems. If we were to eliminate psychiatric testimony, the task of the judge or jury would not be more difficult; rather it would be *easier* because the real evidence of mental intent—the behavior of the accused person—would no longer be confused by psychiatric speculation.

If we exclude psychiatry, how do we deal with those offenders who, defense lawyers say, committed their crimes while in a state of major mental breakdown? There would be, first of all, no recourse to legal insanity as a criminal defense. During the trial, the defense attorney could present evidence showing that the defendant was in a compromised mental state at the time of the crime. The evidence, however, could not include the testimony of psychiatrists or psychologists. Instead, witnesses present during the crime or in contact with the defendant around the time of the crime could testify about what they saw and heard. Any evidence of the defendant's bizarre or irrational behavior would be the subject of proper testimony.

On the basis of this, the judge or jury might decide that even though the individual was seriously impaired, he or she nonetheless intended to kill the victim and is therefore guilty of murder. In another case, the judge or jury might conclude that the defendant's irrational behavior shows he or she had no intent to kill. The person would be guilty of manslaughter, not murder.

The approach to punishment would also be different. No offenders would be indefinitely incarcerated, as they are now. Instead they would be given the definite sentence assigned to their crime, *no more and no less than the person with no mental disorder.* When their sentences expire, they would be released, with no possibility of confinement being extended because of alleged dangerousness. Neither could persons be released sooner than the release date because of alleged restoration of sanity, or because of any "plan of supervision, management, and treatment."

During confinement, no psychiatric treatments could be forced on any person. Instead inmates would be *offered* help, as well as the opportunity to serve their time in a specially staffed and therapeutically oriented prison (we now call these places hospitals for the criminally insane). They would be free to terminate this treatment at any time and return to prison to serve the rest of the sentence.

This plan requires of society the courage to admit that while the plan appears to be "taking a chance" on the mentally disordered offender, definite sentences for all offenders are no more risky (and probably less risky) than what we do now. All along we have been "taking a chance" on psychiatry, believing that its expert examinations would protect us. If we have lived with this false prophecy for so long, certainly we can do as well and probably better without it.

CHAPTER 4

DIMINISHED CAPACITY
Expanding Psychiatry's Courtroom Empire

On the morning of November 27, 1978, Dan White loaded his .38 caliber revolver. Familiar with guns, the former policeman and Vietnam veteran put ten extra hollow point cartridges in his pocket and went to City Hall.

White had recently resigned his position as a San Francisco supervisor because of family and financial pressures. Now, after a change of heart, he wanted his job back. When he asked Mayor George Moscone to reappoint him, however, the mayor refused. Supervisor Harvey Milk was among those who had urged Moscone to keep White out, for Milk was America's first openly gay politician, and Dan White had been an outspoken opponent of measures supporting gay rights.[1]

White avoided the metal detector at City Hall's main entrance by climbing through a basement window after telling construction workers who recognized him that he had forgotten his keys. After they unlocked the window for him, he went straight to the mayor's office. There Moscone greeted him and poured a couple of drinks, perhaps hoping to soothe White's rage at not being reappointed. Neither man had a chance to touch his drink before White pulled out his gun and shot the mayor once in the arm and once in the chest. As Moscone lay bleeding on the floor, White walked over to him and, from only inches away, fired twice more into Moscone's head.

White then reloaded his gun, ran down the hall, and spotted Harvey Milk. White asked to talk with him. Right after the two men went into White's former office, three more shots rang out. Milk crumpled to the floor. Once again White from point-blank range fired two more bullets into his victim's head. After escaping through the same basement window, White walked to his parish church, later calling his wife to meet him there. Shortly afterward he turned himself in to the police. Several months later the jury rendered its verdict: Dan White was not guilty of murder, only voluntary manslaughter.

Murder is the illegal killing of a human being with malice aforethought, that is, with the intent to kill. Manslaughter is the illegal killing of a human being *without* malice aforethought. The attacker may intend to harm the victim, but not to kill. If the victim nonetheless dies, the crime is voluntary manslaughter. Involuntary manslaughter is an illegal killing from negligence rather than intentional harm.

When the jury found White guilty only of voluntary manslaughter, it decided that White did not intend to kill Moscone or Milk. Most San Franciscans reacted with confusion and anger. The decision seemed to lack basic common sense. How could a man who loaded his pistol with cartridges that explode on impact, who made a conscious effort to avoid the metal detector, and who, finally, walked over to the prone, wounded men and shot each one twice more in the head—how could such a man be said to have no murderous intent?

The answer lies in the role psychiatry played in the trial.[2] Defense attorney Douglas Schmidt argued that a patriotic, civic-minded man like Dan White—high school athlete, decorated war veteran, former fireman, policeman, and city supervisor—could not possibly have committed such an act unless something had snapped inside him. The brutal nature of the two final shots to each man's head only proved that White had lost his wits. White was not fully responsible for his actions because he suffered from "diminished capacity." Although White killed Mayor

George Moscone and Supervisor Harvey Milk, he had not planned his actions. On the day of the shootings, White was mentally incapable of planning to kill, or even of wanting to do such a thing.

Schmidt took advantage of the fact that the jury would be instructed by the judge to decide not only whether White had planned the killings but also whether he had planned them with "mature and meaningful" reflection. The judge would also instruct the jury to decide not simply whether White intended to kill his victims but whether he had at that moment "an awareness of an obligation to act within the general body of law regulating society."

Just as important, Schmidt knew that the jury would not decide these questions on the basis of White's overt acts, but would look for guidance from experts in psychiatry. Weeks, even months after his acts, these experts would examine White to determine what he was thinking at the moment of the killings. They would then tell the jury whether or not White was reflecting "meaningfully and maturely" on his acts, whether or not he was aware at that moment of his "obligation to society." The jury might be so taken up with defense and prosecution psychiatrists' claims and counterclaims that the obvious facts at hand might be confused or overlooked entirely. In that ploy lay White's only chance of avoiding conviction for premeditated murder.

The first psychiatrist took the stand. He was Jerry Jones of Stockton. Asked by Schmidt if White had intended to kill Moscone and Milk, Jones replied, "He was just, you know, striking out."[3] Later probed during cross-examination by the assistant district attorney Thomas Norman on whether or not White knew that two shots to the head would kill, Jones was willing to testify, "I don't even think that kind of idea was in his mind."

Schmidt's next expert witness was a man with considerable credentials. Well known in forensic psychiatry circles, Martin Blinder, professor of law and psychiatry at the University of California's Hastings Law School in San Francisco, brought a good measure of academic prestige to White's defense. White had been, Blinder explained to the jury, "gorging himself on junk food: Twinkies, Coca-Cola . . . The more he consumed, the worse he'd feel and he'd respond to his ever-growing depression by consuming ever more junk food." Schmidt later asked Blinder if he could elaborate on this. "Perhaps if it were not for the ingestion of this junk food," Blinder responded, "I would suspect that these homicides would not have taken place." From that moment on, Blinder became known as the author of the Twinkie Defense.

The next psychiatrist, George F. Solomon, further drove home the idea that it was not Dan White but an irritating extraneous influence—something outside himself—that made White do these terrible things. Did White have the capacity to premeditate and deliberate murder? "No," Solomon responded. "Why not?" he was asked. "I don't think that he would permit himself—he was capable of permitting himself to plan something so awful." The killings, Solomon told the jury, were the result of "a dissociated state of mind, which means a disruption of the normal integrated functions." White had, Solomon continued, "blocked out of his mind his awareness of his duty to uphold the right."

Solomon further contended that White did not take the gun with him to City Hall that fateful November day in order to shoot Moscone and Milk. When prosecutor Norman asked Solomon during the cross-examination why White carried the gun, he replied, "The gun was a security blanket in certain ways . . . security blankets are clung to in situations of great anxiety as one sees with children, of course, with the actual teddy bear or the security blanket." Why did White need a security blanket on that particular day? Norman asked. Solomon responded, "I assume that he was more anxious on this occasion than he had been on other occasions when he had been in City Hall."

If White was in such a "dissociated state," Norman asked, how did he have the wits to reload his gun? "He told me," Solomon answered, "that he had been taught to reload a gun after it was discharged." Was White angry as he sought out and killed Supervisor Milk? White was not angry, Solomon said, but was "sort of on automatic pilot."

The next defense expert, psychologist Richard Delman, had given White an inkblot test, an intelligence test, and a personality test. From these he concluded that White had "lived his life by the Golden Rule." White's deep concern for others, Delman explained, led him to sneak into City Hall through a window rather than face the detection of his gun by the metal detector at the front door. According to Delman, White "didn't want to embarrass the officer who was operating the metal detector."

Finally, Schmidt called another psychiatrist of considerable courtroom experience, Donald Lunde of Stanford University. In the days following his crimes, could White have lied to any of his psychiatric examiners? Lunde was asked. No, replied Lunde; he was sure White was not able to "consciously fabricate." Furthermore, Lunde held that White "was literally not focusing . . . his eyes on the Mayor. He was vaguely only aware of the Mayor and of the Mayor falling and the gun going off again." White, in other words, became two beings: Lunde testified, "What was going on was not any series of thinking, but, rather, a reacting to this human form and firing the gun and almost watching himself do it, sort of a state of depersonalization, as you would call it, wherein somebody has the sensation of being almost out of their body and watching themselves do something."

The defense called five experts: four psychiatrists and one psychologist; prosecutor Norman called only one psychiatrist. Norman believed that the murders spoke for themselves. To him, no juror could fail to see that Dan

White had planned these killings. But Norman underestimated two factors: first, the power of psychiatric testimony to compete with common sense, and, second, the confusion that the legal definitions of diminished capacity would present to the jury. It is one thing to decide, as judges and juries did before the concept of diminished capacity came along, whether or not the accused intended to kill the victim, and whether or not the accused did so with advance planning (premeditation). It is quite another thing to decide, after a barrage of psychiatric claims and counterclaims, whether or not the accused "meaningfully and maturely" reflected on his or her acts and whether or not the accused "was aware of an obligation to society."

Dan White was convicted only of voluntary manslaughter, and was sentenced to seven years, eight months. (He was released on parole January 6, 1984.) Psychiatric testimony convinced the jury that White, as he blew each man's brains out, did not wish to kill George Moscone or Harvey Milk.

The angry crowd that responded to the verdict by marching, shouting, trashing City Hall, and burning police cars was in good part homosexual. Gay supervisor Harvey Milk had worked well for their cause, and his loss was a serious setback for human rights in San Francisco. Yet it was not only members of the gay community who were appalled at the outcome. Most San Franciscans shared their feelings of outrage.

What many people failed to recognize was that the powerful role played by psychiatric testimony extended beyond the courtroom itself. The confusing legal terms like "meaningful and mature reflection" were the result of earlier psychiatric influence on our nation's most influential judges.

Defining Diminished Capacity

The Dan White trial illustrates what happens when a diminished capacity defense is successfully presented to a judge or jury. The defense lawyer argues that mental disorder prevented the accused from having the capacity to harbor the mental intent required for this particular crime. If the court accepts this claim, then the person will either be excused completely or, more likely, found guilty only of a lesser crime. For a finding of premeditated murder, the judge or jury must believe that the killer not only intended for the victim to die, but also planned the crime. For a finding of unpremeditated murder, the judge or jury must believe that even though the accused did not plan the killing, he or she did wish to kill at the moment the act was being committed.

People who followed the Dan White trial became enraged at the jury's decision because they believed that the facts clearly pointed to premeditation, deliberation, and full intent to kill. Particularly upsetting was the feeling that if the psychiatrists had not come armed with theories about Twinkies and security blankets, the jury would have seen the facts for what they were. Indeed, before the diminished capacity defense was invented, this was much more often the case. In distinguishing between murder and manslaughter, the judge or jury did not determine a person's *capacity* for criminal intent, based on psychiatrists' opinions about that capacity. Instead they determined a person's intent by looking at the facts: the concrete evidence surrounding the crime, particularly the behavior of the accused.[4] A review of how this new and confusing approach was developed and used by lawyers and psychiatrists will show why we need a return to a more traditional approach.

Proud Confessions from Law

In the months following the White trial, attorney Douglas Schmidt was a much sought-after man: He was asked to lecture and appear on panels to explain how he had won what seemed like an impossible verdict. Lawyers were particularly curious about this feat. They knew that Schmidt had received unintentional help from the opposition: An inept prosecution team had chosen to play for the jury a tape-recording of White's tearful confession. Instead of convincing the jury that White was guilty of murder, the tape brought several members of the jury to tears themselves and undoubtedly encouraged a sympathetic verdict. Lawyers also knew that the prosecution team had only called in one psychiatrist, not enough to counteract the testimony of Schmidt's five experts. What lawyers didn't know was how Schmidt had coaxed out of his five experts the sworn statements about Twinkies and Coca-Cola, death by automatic pilot, and eyes that did not focus. Now they found out.

At the National Homicide Symposium in October, 1979, Schmidt openly described how he did it.

> After you have several psychiatrists examine the defendant, you begin lobbying them . . . going to psychiatrist A and saying, "well, give me some idea of what you think, did he have the capacity for harboring malice and premeditation?" And he's equivocal. He says, "Well, uh, possibly, but uh, you know, I haven't really come to any determination."
>
> Well then, embellishing on that just a bit, you go to psychiatrist B and say, "Well, I talked to psychiatrist A and, perhaps overstating it just a bit, uh, he thinks that probably there isn't too much of the capacity for deliberation and premeditation. I think probably he feels that at the time of the crime the defendant could not harbor these mental states." Psychiatrist B more often than not will say, "Well, I tend to agree with that." Well then, I think you can state a stronger position to the third one and so on. In other words, working one opinion against another until you come down to a refined position.

At the very least, these tactics seem unethical, but they are remarkably revealing. Schmidt could never have manipulated his psychiatrists in this manner *if psychiatrists had means to scientifically determine White's past mental states.* Whereas other medical doctors base their findings on scientific data, such as X-rays or blood tests, psychiatrists base their so-called findings only on subjective evaluations and personal opinions. Schmidt could never have escalated or embellished bona fide medical findings, as he did with the opinions of the psychiatrists.

The most important lesson of Schmidt's proud confession, thus, is this: Psychiatrists are no more able to determine diminished capacity than legal insanity. Interestingly, the person most instrumental in designing and implementing the diminished capacity defense, psychiatrist Bernard Diamond, was one of the first to admit this.

Proud Confessions from Psychiatry

Professor of psychiatry at the University of California and professor of law at the prestigious Boalt Hall of Law, Bernard Diamond can be called the father of the diminished capacity defense. As we saw in the previous chapter, psychiatry by the 1950s and 1960s was pushing hard to expand the role of the psychiatrist in the courtroom. If psychiatric testimony on legal insanity was frequently confusing, the leaders of forensic psychiatry argued, this was only because psychiatry wasn't allowed to go far enough. The "right-wrong" test for insanity (M'Naughten test) was too limiting. Psychiatrists should get into the courtroom in greater, rather than fewer numbers, and testify on wider considerations than right and wrong. This would require either a broader definition of legal insanity, or a whole new concept of criminal responsibility that would allow psychiatrists to testify even when an insanity defense had *not* been raised.

Today, *both* of these ideas have been embodied in law. First, more and more states now allow psychiatrists to testify not only on whether the accused knew right from wrong but also on whether he or she was impelled to commit the crime by an "irresistible impulse." Second, psychiatry succeeded in carving out an even wider role for the courtroom psychiatrist, through the diminished capacity defense. Two persons were most instrumental in bringing about this development: Lawyer Charles Garry and psychiatrist Bernard Diamond.

Backed by the approval or acquiescence of psychiatry's leading figures, Diamond was so convinced that his campaign for "diminished responsibility" was the correct approach that he was willing to testify to things he knew to be untrue. Because he and his colleagues so strongly disagreed with the prevailing rules governing psychiatric testimony, they felt they had every right to stretch the truth.

Why am I willing to make such serious accusations? Because Diamond has admitted as much in his own writings. In the *Stanford Law Review* in 1961, for example, he discussed his testimony on behalf of a woman who had killed her child.[5] Diamond wrote that he believed that "she knew the nature and quality of her act and that it was wrong." She was, in other words, legally sane under current California law. Nonetheless, Diamond withheld this opinion from the court. "There was no difficulty," he wrote, "in convincing the court that the defendant was legally insane and did not know right from wrong."[6]

This kind of behavior on the witness stand constitutes a criminal act (perjury) and represents a violation of professional ethics. Psychiatry's leaders, with Diamond in the forefront, knew this well. But if the law itself could be changed, allowing psychiatrists more leeway, they could speculate to their hearts' content without having to resort to such tactics. Indeed Diamond said in the same article, "This perjury can be justified and explained away by all sorts of rationalizations . . . but I don't like taking refuge in such semantic devices."[7] The solution, Diamond argued, was the concept of diminished responsibility. No longer restricted to whether the accused person knew right from wrong, the psychiatrist would be much freer to explain the defendant's thinking to the court. This would help criminal courts catch up with modern psychiatric thinking, and also advance the cause of justice.

Has this in fact happened? The Dan White verdict hardly supports these claims. But perhaps that trial was the exception. Let us look at some other trials, starting with those that opened up this new arena for psychiatric testimony.

The Trial of Robert Wesley Wells

One day in 1949, after having already served twenty-one years in California prisons, Robert Wesley Wells was called before a disciplinary hearing in the office of the warden of Folsom State Prison. Wells had been involved in an angry dispute with a guard. Once in the warden's office, Wells soon became enraged at the proceeding and the warden dismissed him summarily. Outside the hearing room, several guards tried to quiet him down. Another argument ensued, and this time Wells threw a cuspidor at one of the guards, the same one he had argued with earlier. The cuspidor broke the guard's jaw.[8]

Wells was charged with assault and eventually found guilty. Because he, like so many other California prisoners, was already serving an indeterminate sentence with a maximum of life imprisonment, the death penalty could be invoked. This was because a draconian California law (now fortunately repealed) said that any prisoner serving a "life sentence" (even if it was a sentence of six months to life for a nonviolent crime) who assaulted a guard "with malice aforethought" could be put to death.[9] Wells was thus scheduled to die in the gas chamber.

Wells' attorneys appealed this conviction to the California Supreme Court. They did not claim he was legally insane. It was too late for that. Rather they argued that Wells should not get the death penalty because when he threw the cuspidor, he did not act with malice. Because of his emotional turmoil, they argued, he did not really know what he was doing. Today this is not an unusual defense. But at that time it was unheard of outside of insanity trials. Unless a defendant claimed to be legally insane—and Wells had not done this—psychiatrists could not testify about a defendant's mental state. Now, before California's highest court, Wells' attorneys argued that the testimony of the prison doctors, who claimed Wells was emotionally distraught, should have been heard at his trial. His attorneys argued that expert opinions regarding Wells' state of mind would have helped the trial court decide whether Wells did or did not have malice aforethought.

The California Supreme Court did not overturn Wells' conviction. Significantly, however, it did agree with the lawyers' arguments about psychiatric testimony. The court ruled that from then on such testimony was admissible in the courtroom even without a plea of insanity. This ruling was an important first step in expanding the use of courtroom psychiatry, but it still left Bob Wells facing the death penalty. Thus, an appeal to the United States Supreme Court was prepared, and lawyer Charles Garry then entered the case. It was at this point that Garry and Diamond began formulating their plan, one that would clearly establish a greater role for psychiatric testimony in the courtroom and eventually become the diminished capacity defense.

As it turned out, the United States Supreme Court refused to hear Wells' appeal.[10] Fortunately, however, Wells was not sent to the gas chamber. His death sentence was later commuted to life imprisonment by California's governor.

The ruling that psychiatrists could testify in California courts on whether or not the accused acted with criminal intent, even if legal insanity was not being claimed, did not at first bring significant change. The ruling did not take full effect until 1957, when a San Francisco dockworker killed his boss.

The Landmark Case of Nicholas Gorshen

It was not until ten years after the *Wells* case that psychiatrist Diamond and lawyer Garry saw their efforts bear fruit. In another decision by the California Supreme Court, the door was opened wide for the possible entry of psychiatry into virtually all trials for serious crimes.[11] The case that resulted in this drastic expansion of courtroom psychiatry was the murder trial of Nicholas Gorshen.

Nicholas Gorshen emigrated to the United States from Russia in 1923. He got a job as a longshoreman on the docks of San Francisco and stayed there until March 8, 1957, the day he shot and killed his boss. On that fateful day, Gorshen got so drunk on his lunch break that his boss, Red O'Leary, ordered him to go home and sleep it off. When Gorshen refused, O'Leary soundly thrashed him. Gorshen became so outraged that he yelled to everyone nearby that he was going home to get his gun and would return to kill O'Leary. Because he seemed angry enough to carry out his threat, his fellow workers called the police. When Gorshen returned to the docks, the police were waiting for him. They searched him thoroughly, but somehow failed to find his gun. As they were about to leave, Gorshen quickly drew his pistol and fired a lethal shot into O'Leary.

Enter Garry and Diamond. Since the *Wells* case, this team had been waiting for a case to emerge that would give them the opportunity to establish firmly their new doctrine of "diminished responsibility." Despite the ruling in the *Wells* case, psychiatrists were still only being called to court when an insanity defense was presented. Garry and Diamond believed more cases must demonstrate the need for psychiatry in the courtroom, even when there was no apparent evidence of serious mental disorder. Ever since the *Wells* case, they, along with lawyer Benjamin Dreyfus, had continued to work together on (to quote Diamond) "the possibilities for this type of psychiatric testimony."[12] As Diamond later wrote,

> The trial of Nicholas Gorshen was carefully planned from the very beginning to utilize to the fullest possible extent psychiatric evidence to disprove premeditation and malice aforethought . . . When Nicholas Gorshen shot and killed his longshoreman boss, the lawyers and the psychiatrists, so to speak, were ready and waiting for him.[13]

A brief look at the trial itself will indicate what Diamond meant. Numerous eyewitnesses testified that they had not only seen Gorshen kill his boss but also heard Gorshen shout his earlier threats. Gorshen confessed to the crime and never once claimed he did not know what he was doing. A conviction of premeditated murder seemed inevitable.[14]

Nevertheless Diamond in his testimony contradicted the observable facts by claiming that Gorshen's state of mind at the time of the killing prevented him from either intending to kill or premeditating the crime. According to Diamond, Gorshen went into a trance when he committed the murder. In an article written after the trial, the same one in which he openly spoke of committing perjury in insanity trials, Diamond said:

> When I examined Gorshen *there was little or no evidence of mental illness.* But I was alerted by two facts: One, that the crime was completely out of keeping with the defendant's previous personality; and two, that his nickname had been for many years "Sleepy." Out of these simple clues there developed a strange and fascinating story of a *secret mental illness which had never before been*

revealed to even his closest friends or family . . . he had had these sleepy spells for at least 20 years, perhaps once or twice a week . . . during those few moments of trance, he entered into a strange world populated by demons, strange animals, and bizarre and deformed people [emphasis added].[15]

Gorshen totally denied these things were taking place. Even Diamond later admitted this, writing that Gorshen "was frank in stating that he was not in a trance when he quarreled with or killed O'Leary. He claimed he knew full well what he was doing and very deliberately planned to kill."[16]

Garry and Diamond were not about to accept Gorshen's willingness to take full responsibility for his act. They pushed on. In his sworn testimony Diamond told the court that Gorshen was a chronic paranoid schizophrenic. As such, Gorshen was forced by the fist fight to confront

the imminent possibility of complete loss of his sanity . . . An individual in this state of crisis will do anything to avoid the threatened insanity . . . The shooting itself released the danger of defendant's complete mental disintegration.[17]

This insistence that Gorshen was a "schizophrenic" is hard to square with Diamond's later statement that "there was little or no evidence of mental illness."

This testimony produced a verdict of second-degree murder rather than of first-degree (premeditated) murder. Hoping to reduce the verdict even further, to voluntary manslaughter, Garry presented an appeal to the California Supreme Court. The court did not reverse the lower court's decision, but nonetheless completely swallowed Diamond's claims. The court wrote:

The doctor [Diamond] further explained that in his opinion, "actions like the threat to kill, the going home to get the gun and so forth"—actions which "in an ordinary individual" would be evidence "that he intended to do what he did do and that this was an act of free will and deliberation"—in defendant's case were rather "just as much symptoms of his mental illness as the visions and these trances that he goes into."[18]

One of the most influential courts in the nation was saying that in a battle between common sense and psychiatry, common sense should lose. During this appeal, eighteen of psychiatry's biggest names filed a brief urging that this kind of psychiatric testimony be accepted as the norm.[19] Only through the testimony on Gorshen's mental state, they argued, had the court been given "an explanation of the criminal act, which otherwise was inexplicable." Diamond, they continued, "followed basic principles of psychiatry and law established by the most authoritative textbooks in the field."[20]

These statements were written by psychiatry's leaders, representing thousands of their lesser-known colleagues. It was perfectly acceptable to testify about "secret" mental illnesses and about trances that even the accused person denied. All this was "authoritative" and essential in a court of law.

Talking with Nicholas Gorshen

Twenty years after his famous trial I was able to locate Mr. Gorshen, living in San Francisco. Paroled from prison after five years, he had resumed living with his wife until her death in 1979. He was now nearing eighty years of age, yet he was still alert. When I explained that I was a psychiatrist and had a special interest in his trial, he was quite friendly and willing to talk.

He had no idea his case had set a legal precedent. He couldn't recall what Diamond had said about him at the trial, although he did remember several interviews before the trial. I reminded him of Diamond's testimony about trances and demons, and that Diamond had labeled him a chronic paranoid schizophrenic. Gorshen had not only forgotten all this; he didn't believe Diamond's claims.

When I asked if he was in a trance when he shot O'Leary, Gorshen smiled and said, "No, I never thought of anything like that." He did remember telling Diamond of daydreams he had had during periods of idleness. "They were kind of images of what life should be like," he said. "They came on when I was drowsy or not doing much. They'd just last for a few minutes, then go away. Nothing special." I asked about daydreams on the day of the crime. "No," he said, "they didn't come that day and they had nothing to do with the killing." He said he had no idea that these daydreams had been magnified into a "secret mental illness."

I reminded Gorshen of the testimony that mental illness had forced him to kill his boss, that the killing protected him from a full-blown schizophrenic break with reality. At this Gorshen laughed. He said he would like to read more about the trial. Until now, he had not paid much attention to the psychiatric testimony.

"What took place that day?" I asked him. He responded that he and several others had taken an extra long lunch break and had had too much to drink. This was not unusual among the dockworkers, but his boss was not the sort to avoid a confrontation. "I didn't really like the man because he was always bragging about how tough he was." After they had argued and O'Leary had easily knocked him down, Gorshen was not only angry but humiliated. He yelled his murderous threats and went home to get his gun. When he returned with the gun, he wasn't sure if he would use it.

After the police searched me, O'Leary was laughing at me. The police told me to go home. I got in my car and almost drove off but O'Leary was still laughing. I was twenty or thirty feet away, and I thought, "That's gonna be his last laugh."

Gorshen fired a single shot. O'Leary was hit in the thigh and did not appear seriously hurt, but a few hours later he died.

As he told me the story, Gorshen at no time made even the vaguest mention of demons, trances, or any other altered states of mind. He made no excuses for his crime. He frankly admitted that the killing was a matter of plain stupidity on his part and he accepted full responsibility for it. Had he ever received any psychiatric treatment while in prison? I asked. "No," he said. "I had no need for it and none of the doctors thought so either." No one but Diamond had ever seen or heard of Gorshen's "secret mental illness."

The Impact of the Gorshen Case

Gorshen's trial is significant for one main reason: California's highest court ruled that the role of psychiatry in criminal trials would now be expanded. Since California is considered a judicial and legal trend-setter, the other states noted well that psychiatrists could now be called to testify about whether a defendant possessed criminal intent at the time of a crime, even though a defense of insanity was not entered.

This was the birth of the diminished capacity defense, just as Diamond and Garry had planned it years earlier. And if we again consult his own writings, it is clear that Diamond knew perfectly well that a few tricks were being played.

> I concede that this whole business of lack of mental capacity to premeditate, to have malice or entertain intent, is a kind of sophistry . . . *we must utilize these legal technicalities to permit the psychiatrists to gain entrance into the trial court* . . .

the next step . . . is to expand the principle of limited or diminished responsibility of the mentally
ill offender to include *all definitions of crime* [em-
phasis added].[21]

Two decades later, most states have incorporated this
"sophistry" into their criminal trial procedures.[22]

Redefining Diminished Capacity

Since the Gorshen trial, things have gone from bad to
worse. Precisely what the psychiatrists are supposed to be
telling the judge or jury about the accused's mental state
has become less and less clear. On the surface of things,
psychiatrists are supposed to be telling the court about the
criminal intent an accused did or did not harbor at the
time of the crime. In a murder trial, for example, the question is whether the person intended to kill the victim and
if so whether it was a premeditated murder or an impul-
sive act.

But the term *criminal intent*, with psychiatry's help,
has become so convoluted that law professor Phillip Johnson claims it makes sense only to a "medieval scholastic
theologian."[23] Similarly, law professor Peter Arenella has
written that the diminished capacity defense asks a jury
"to make distinctions worthy of a medieval schoolmas-
ter."[24] What Johnson and Arenella mean is that the diminished capacity defense enlarged the question of "intent to
kill" to include "an awareness of the obligation to act
within the general body of laws regulating society."[25]
Again, *premeditation* has traditionally meant simply
"advance planning." But the diminished capacity defense
required also that the accused person "maturely and meaningfully reflected upon the gravity of his contemplated
act."[26] Finally, Johnson and Arenella refer to the fact that
courts traditionally used the facts of the case to decide,
without help from psychiatry, whether the accused person

did or did not intend to kill and did or did not plan it beforehand. With the diminished capacity defense, courts must decide whether the accused had the *capacity* to harbor these things in his or her mind.

As a result, a psychiatrist may testify that while the manner in which the crime was committed might *seem* to show criminal intent, mental illness prohibited that person from in fact having that criminal intent. Thus, Diamond could testify in the *Gorshen* case that "actions like the threat to kill" might show premeditation in an "ordinary individual." But in someone who a psychiatrist decided was not "ordinary" and was "mentally ill," those very same actions would *not* show premeditation or malice.

Through these developments, psychiatry has indeed carved out a new role for itself. More and more criminal trials, not just murder trials, have become forums for psychiatric speculations. As prosecuting attorney Dino Fulgoni has said, "Seldom does a serious criminal case filter through the courts of California without the appointment of at least two psychiatrists to determine whether the defense of diminished capacity is a viable possibility."[27]

Because I frequently testify in criminal trials that the judge or jury should give no weight to psychiatric opinions concerning mental intent—and I offer none myself—I have had a chance to read the reports and hear the testimony of many psychiatrists and psychologists. What I have seen again and again is that the kind of testimony given in the trials of Dan White and Nicholas Gorshen is commonplace; it occurs almost every time psychiatry enters the courtroom for trials involving violent and nonviolent crimes alike. And it makes no difference whether the testifying psychiatrists are recent graduates or well-established figures. Sometimes even the one who stands to gain from the testimony finds it difficult to swallow.

Inez Garcia Speaks Her Mind

In March 1974, Inez Garcia was raped by two men in Soledad, California. After the ordeal was finally over, she ran home, got her rifle, and went looking for them. Six bullets later, Miguel Jimenez was dead and Inez Garcia faced charges of first-degree murder.

The trial became a *cause célèbre* for the radical feminist movement, and the courtroom was packed with women who believed Inez Garcia was justified in what she did. But under the law she had no right to kill her attackers, since it was not an act of immediate self-defense. Attorney Charles Garry was retained, and he called psychiatrist Jane Olden to testify about the state of Inez Garcia's mind when she evened the score.

Olden testified that the rape had provoked in Garcia an impaired consciousness or sleepwalking state. As a result she did not really know what she was doing. On cross-examination, Olden elaborated:

> In her particular kind of condition, if you trigger off negative feelings about herself which are primarily unconscious and covered over by these reactive formations of being concerned about children's welfare and, you know, what I term a saint-like idealized virgin, if you trigger her into negative feelings, which would be provoked by such an act as rape, being a hysterical person who was striving always to suppress this sensuality and aggression, then you could indeed throw her into a state where she is emotionally relating to her own inner conflict . . . what I am saying is when you say she was excited, she was unquestionably at a very high level of energy and anxiety and tension or whatever, excitement, but mostly because of the threat to her inner psyche conflicts is what I'm trying to get across, so she blocked out her best judgment or

what is right in the eyes of society and she takes it upon herself to defend herself.[28]

One can only guess what Inez Garcia thought of these comments, but just a few moments later she jumped up from the counsel table, pushed her way to the judge's bench, and yelled, "I killed the motherfucker because I was raped and I'd kill him again. You're acting like . . ." Before she could finish, she was dragged from the courtroom.

Abolishing Diminished Capacity

Like the insanity defense, the diminished capacity defense hinders the judge or jurors in their determinations of criminal intent. It does so by substituting psychiatric guesswork for real evidence. It should be discarded. The alternative is to simply let the judge or jurors decide questions of criminal intent as they did before psychiatry introduced the confusion seen in trials from Nicholas Gorshen to Dan White. A defendant should be allowed to claim a lack of intent and introduce evidence to support the claim, but not be permitted to use psychiatric testimony. Next, legislators should spell out clear and simple definitions of *premeditation* and *malice*. Before psychiatry came into these trials, *premeditation* meant "advance planning," and *malice* meant "the intent to kill." We should return to these simple and straightforward definitions.

With a return to common-sense legal definitions, and with a ban on psychiatric testimony, the diminished capacity defense would be eliminated. A court would no longer ask whether a defendant had the *capacity* to harbor a specific criminal intent. Instead, the facts of the case would indicate whether the accused *did or did not* have a specific intent. Society would no longer be burdened with—and be expected to pay for—trials in which the facts indicate that criminal intent was present, while psychiatrists testify that the defendant nonetheless did not have the *capacity* to intend to do what he or she obviously did intend to do. If Dan White, for example, did not intend to kill George Moscone and Harvey Milk, he would not have put his gun against each man's skull and fired two bullets into each man's brain.

Those found to have committed a crime with the required intent would be found guilty and sentenced accordingly. Those found guilty of a lesser crime (for example, manslaughter rather than murder), because the prosecution could not prove the more serious intent, would be sentenced to the penalty prescribed for the lesser crime.

In 1981 the California legislature took an important step in this direction. No longer do judges and juries in that state need to ask whether an accused person planned the crime "meaningfully and maturely," only whether the accused planned it. No longer do they ask whether the accused person killed the victim while having an "awareness of his obligation to society," only whether the person intended to kill.

The California legislature did not remove psychiatry from these trials and the new law is only a single step, but it is an important first step. Psychiatric testimony, and the fuzzy definitions designed to promote psychiatric testimony, should be banned from criminal trials.

CHAPTER 5

INCOMPETENT TO STAND TRIAL
Guilty until Proven Innocent

The insanity defense makes headlines in trials like that of John Hinckley, but there is a much more common and less publicized way by which psychiatry clouds and confuses our criminal courts. Solely on the basis of psychiatric opinion, a criminal defendant may be ruled incompetent to stand trial. Criminal charges are then suspended while the person is sent to a mental institution. When the person has received enough treatment to enable him or her to understand the criminal charges and to rationally assist the defense lawyer, the trial will proceed. The purpose is to make sure the accused gets a fair trial. That, at least, is the theory.

In practice our courts are using psychiatry in competency hearings more out of convenience than from any consideration of justice.[1] In case after case fundamental rights are denied by maneuvers for competency rulings. In some cases it is the accused person's constitutional right to a speedy trial that is denied. In other cases it is the right of the people to hold criminals responsible for their acts that is denied. Let us see how this happens.

A Matter of Convenience

The concerns behind a hearing to determine incompetence for trial seem sound, but the real motivation for these hearings is often very different. Quite regularly, all the participants ignore the laws regulating this issue. They find persons incompetent for reasons that have nothing to do with the defendant's ability to understand criminal charges or to assist his lawyer.[2] Psychiatrist Abraham Halpern has written of the

> tendency shown by the principals in the court world—judge, prosecutor, and defense attorney— to serve their individual and separate ends by involving the psychiatrist, who is sometimes quite readily available but almost always unsuspecting of his inappropriate use or blatant misuse.[3]

What are the motives behind this practice? Sometimes, the prosecutor uses this method to get the accused locked up (in a mental institution) without having to prove the person guilty of any crime.[4] Sometimes the defense attorney uses this method in the hope that the prosecutor will drop criminal charges. Sometimes this approach serves as a preliminary ploy in building a case based on a plea of legal insanity. Sometimes a judge uses this device to clear a court calendar of a case quickly and conveniently, or to satisfy the will of the community by confining deviant persons in mental hospitals longer than the civil commitment process will allow.

Psychiatrist Ralph Slovenko, in *Psychiatry and Law*, has written:

> Quite frequently the prosecuting attorney or the judge raises the issue of the accused's unfitness to proceed so as to accomplish the goal of preventive or long-term detention, which otherwise could not be available under the criminal law process. The criminal charge serves as little more than a fictional jurisdictional excuse for indeterminate confinement.[5]

This hardly adds up to being "fair." But what specifically is going wrong? Henry Steadman, of the New York Department of Mental Hygiene, recently studied how psychiatrists, judges, and lawyers determine if a person is unfit to stand trial.[6] He examined the cases of 539 people declared incompetent after being hospitalized in a New York City psychiatric ward. Most of these inmates were nonwhite and more than half had not even been formally indicted for a crime.

The typical hearing, which took place in the hospital day room, where a few chairs had been arranged, took two to three minutes. If the psychiatrist found the person to be incompetent, the judge rubber-stamped this opinion. "The defendants," Steadman found, "were often on psychotropic medications and were not in touch with much of what was going on around them."[7] In about one-third of the cases the person contested the psychiatrist's report; the hearing in this instance took longer—about twenty minutes. Especially noteworthy was that in most cases it was the prosecuting attorney, not the defense attorney, who sought a finding of incompetence. Steadman pointed out the convenience of this arrangement: "It can represent an easy way out for the district attorney and the state. They get the person off the street for an indefinite time in a maximum security facility without criminal prosecution."[8]

In my own experience, even when the defense attorney calls for a competency hearing, the reason usually has more to do with psychiatric maneuvering than any real indication that the accused is unable to understand the charges or assist a lawyer. The Group for the Advancement of Psychiatry studied competency hearings, and described the defense tactics as "a device to delay trial, whether because they believe delay will help their case, or because delay offers the busy lawyer a welcome postponement."[9]

In some cases the defense lawyer may merely be preparing for an insanity defense. A finding of incompetence, followed by hospitalization, makes a later insanity defense more likely to succeed. When the trial finally takes place, the reports of hospital psychiatrists can be admitted into evidence, and the very existence of the reports will favor a finding of insanity. The court may well consider any treatments given during the period of hospitalization as proof that the defendant was so mentally ill that he or she lacked criminal responsibility. This reasoning may explain attorney F. Lee Bailey's attempt to have Patricia Hearst found incompetent for trial. There wasn't the slightest indication that she didn't know exactly what was going on, but Bailey knew that her defense would rest on psychiatric testimony, and a prior finding of incompetence would enhance the impact of that testimony.[10] He was not able to convince the judge of his claims, but in less highly publicized cases the same tactics often do work.

It is not unusual for a defense lawyer to assume that placement of the client in a mental institution as incompetent, followed later by a plea of legal insanity, is better for the client than proceeding to trial and risking a guilty verdict. The defendant may strongly disagree, especially if he or she has previously spent time in a mental institution: The client may prefer to go to trial and either be found guilty and sent to prison or be found not guilty and set free. The defense lawyer may sometimes override the person's wishes.

Let us consider, for example, the case of a man I shall call Steve. In 1980 I reviewed his case in consultation with Sanford Svetcov, the U.S. attorney in San Francisco. Earlier, a psychiatrist at the Chester, Illinois, Security Hospital had pronounced Steve incompetent even though he was, according to the psychiatrist's own report, "at present rationally able to understand the nature of the proceedings." Why did the psychiatrist find the man incompetent? The defendant, he said, would not give in to his lawyer's desire for a plea of insanity. Persisting in his refusal to plead insanity, the defendant was found incompetent for trial, over his protests that he wanted to stand trial. He was kept at a mental institution for several years, until he finally agreed to plead insanity. Only then was he promptly found "competent" by hospital psychiatrists. Next, in a twenty-minute hearing he was first certified by the judge as legally competent to stand trial and then certified by the judge as not guilty by reason of insanity. The defendant's reward for his lawyer's persistence? He was sent back to the same mental hospital for more years. The only difference now was his label: Instead of being labeled "incompetent to stand trial," he was now labeled "criminally insane."

The Psychiatrist's Motivation

Psychiatrists making a determination of possible incompetence for trial have a difficult time dealing with the legal issues before them. Instead of focusing on whether or not the defendant can understand the charges and assist an attorney, the psychiatrists concentrate on whether or not they believe the defendant might benefit from psychiatric hospitalization. If they feel the person would benefit, a finding of incompetence will be made, even though the person is quite capable of going on trial and may very much want to do so.[11] This conclusion can be reached by anyone who reviews records of these hearings. An example involving three psychiatrists, instead of one, will clarify this point.

The three doctors worked for the San Diego Mental Health Services and were asked in 1976 to examine a 19-year-old man facing a charge of armed robbery. He had robbed a market at gunpoint. After describing the events of the crime, the defendant's current mental state, and his background, the report concluded, "The patient is still seriously ill. In his present state he represents a danger to the community. He needs continued care."

That was it. Nowhere in the report did the psychiatrists *even mention* the legally relevant question—whether or not the man could understand the charge against him, or could rationally assist his lawyer. Instead, the doctors decided it was their duty to protect society from someone unpleasant, disordered, and dangerous, and their prerogative to decide how to do this. They pronounced him incompetent for trial because this would accomplish what they wanted—mandatory hospitalization. While the psychiatrists may have felt they were answering to a higher authority, the fact remains that they were taking the law into their own hands like vigilantes.

It is disquieting that psychiatrists should disregard the law in this way. It is even more disquieting that courts seldom challenge this lawlessness. Judges, in general, are as guilty as psychiatrists of ignoring the provisions of the law in order to dispose of a case quickly and easily.

I do not make these charges lightly. Many other researchers have reached the same conclusions. Steadman, for example, has written, "It is quite possible to be mentally ill and be competent to stand trial. However, this possibility is usually not recognized or accepted by judges."[12] Psychiatry, pretending to help, has just as often denied mentally disordered persons, as well as perfectly rational persons, their basic legal rights.

One-Way Ticket

After a person is found incompetent to stand trial, he or she is placed in a mental institution, supposedly for treatment that will restore competence. Once in that institution, however, this goal is easily forgotten. For decades, no one bothered to find out what happened to those who were sent to mental institutions because they were incompetent for trial. When several teams of researchers finally ventured inside the hospitals, in the 1960s, what they found wasn't pretty. In Massachusetts, for example, there were "commitments dating back to all but the first decade of the twentieth century. Prior to 1960, only a handful of men committed . . . had ever been returned to trial."[13]

Trying to explain why people were incarcerated for years or decades longer than if they had been found guilty and sent to prison, and sometimes for the rest of their lives, investigators found that institutional psychiatrists showed "a bias against returning men to trial, particularly when the man was regarded as dangerous." They also found that "psychiatrists view trial and possible incarceration as punitive, stressful, antitherapeutic, and destructive; whereas hospitalization is seen as supportive, therapeutic, protective, and enlightened."[14]

When these investigators looked a little deeper, however, they found that the "hospital good, prison bad" rationale related more to the concerns of the psychiatrists than to the health of the patients. Doctors did not want to send a person back to court because if he or she were subsequently released and went on to perform a violent act, the doctor might be blamed. Here is how the researchers put it:

> The spectre of headlines, reporting a "former mental patient" committing a dreadful act of violence weighs heavily. Fear of malpractice suits and of adverse publicity and criticism undoubtedly accounts for the cautious attitude exhibited by many in the profession.[15]

Once a person was locked away, the Massachusetts researchers concluded, "the question relative to competency was neither asked by the court nor was it answered by the hospital." The result, they found, was "indefinite commitment," based on a psychiatric label rather than ability to understand criminal charges. Did the courts protest? To the contrary, "the psychiatric opinions had not been challenged by the courts."[16]

Should anyone be tempted to believe that this situation was unique to Massachusetts, the findings at Pennsylvania's Farview State Hospital were equally bleak. The researchers observed staff conferences that considered whether an inmate had regained his competence for trial and found that

> there was no discussion of the patient's ability to confer with counsel or understand the nature of the proceedings against him. The staff reached a conclusion that the patient was incompetent because they feared he was close to a psychotic breakdown . . . One psychologist explained to me that the patient was unfit to stand trial because he was still too dangerous to be allowed on the streets.[17]

Farview doctors were ignoring the law, as were the doctors in Massachusetts. It is a national pattern.

A few years ago, S. L. Stebel wrote a brilliant account of a man caught in the kind of trap the researchers found in Farview and elsewhere. Stebel's book is called *The Shoe Leather Treatment* because the guards wore boots and did not hesitate to use a few well-placed kicks to help bring their "patients" into line.[18] Bill Thomas, whom I have come to know personally and respect highly, is the subject of the book. He spent nine years at Farview after being found incompetent for trial on charges of assault.

At first, Thomas was a model inmate. He knew that he was capable of going to trial and wanted to do so. He preferred whatever punishment he might receive to indefinite confinement in a mental asylum. It was a long time before he even talked to a mental health professional, but finally he was seen by a psychologist. This, he felt, would surely lead to a transfer back to jail to stand trial. Here is Thomas, sharing the good news with an older inmate, one who knew the ropes better.

> "I was tested today," I said, "by the psychologist Sweet. That's a good sign, don't you think?" I asked.
>
> "Of what?" Willy said, not even looking up.

"That they're thinking of letting me out," I said.

"Now what gives you that idea?" he said.

"Why else would they test me?" I said. "They can see I'm not like most of the others, the tests are to kind of, you know, confirm that."

"The tests are just part of the game to hold you," Willy said. "The tests are to prepare you for staff. That way if you petition the court to get out they have papers to show they examined you. Papers to show you're crazy."

"What if the papers don't show that?" I demanded. Willy sighed. "Man, they can interpret those papers any way they want, don't you know that?" he said.[19]

Competence Through Shock Treatment

Sometimes psychiatry has a truly macabre impact, as it did in the case of Thomas Spychala.[20] Accused of murder, Spychala was found incompetent to stand trial by a California court on February 29, 1968, because each of two psychiatrists appointed by the court offered testimony that he was unable to comprehend the charges against him. The fact that he had on several occasions discussed the events of the alleged crime in a clear manner with both police and his attorney was not sufficient to counteract this psychiatric testimony. Particularly important in light of what happened later was that Spychala never claimed he could not remember the events surrounding the killing. All he ever claimed was that he was innocent.

Sent to Atascadero State Hospital on March 12, 1968, Spychala was forced to undergo thirty-two shock treatments during a two-month period. Just as one would expect from these treatments, Spychala then had difficulty recalling events of the preceding months, including the crucial time of the alleged murder. Nonetheless, he was later declared competent to stand trial on the charges, even though *the treatment (shock) for his "incompetence" was the very thing that compromised his memory.* At the trial he testified that since the shock treatment, he could not remember the events surrounding the murder. The association between shock treatment and loss of memory was flatly denied by the doctor who ordered (but did not administer) the shock treatment, even though memory loss for events in the months preceding shock is well known.

Perhaps it was more than the supervising doctor could bear to admit that the treatment for Spychala's supposed inability to understand the charges had instead compromised this ability. The doctor who actually administered the shock treatment, on the other hand, had no difficulty believing that memory loss had resulted from the shock. It was, in fact, part of the treatment. "It would be a benefit," he stated, "to have some memories forgotten permanently." When asked later whether shock treatment, with its known effects on memory, might interfere with, instead of improve, a person's ability to defend himself in a trial, the doctor responded that he had "never stopped to consider" the matter.

Mr. Spychala, by the way, was found guilty of murder.

The Supreme Court Switches Labels

Because it finally became obvious to nearly everyone that a finding of incompetent to stand trial too often was anything but "fair," the Supreme Court attempted to confront the problem in 1972. The case of *Jackson v. Indiana* involved a twenty-seven-year-old, mentally retarded deaf-mute who on two occasions had stolen four dollars and five dollars from women. Found incompetent to stand trial, he was committed to an asylum indefinitely.[21]

Like all others found incompetent for trial, Jackson was supposedly being held in the asylum until doctors there decided he was mentally fit to return to court and face trial. But like most of those judged incompetent, he was never returned for trial. The fact that Jackson was mentally retarded made it especially clear that doctors would never consider him sufficiently "improved" to stand trial. His commitment, then, amounted to a life sentence for two thefts totaling less than ten dollars.

When the Supreme Court handed down its decision in Jackson's case, it finally acknowledged that thousands of persons were being subjected to an injustice. The Court wrote of "data available which tends to show that many defendants committed before trial [found incompetent] are never tried." The Court also noted, in admittedly muted language, that the promise of "treatment" was hollow. They wrote of "substantial doubts about whether the rationale for pretrial commitment—that care or treatment will aid the accused in attaining competency—is empirically valid given the state of most of our mental institutions." The Court was saying, in a nice way, that these people were being warehoused for life. To right this wrong, the Court ordered that henceforth

> a person charged by a State with a criminal offense who is committed solely on account of his incapacity to proceed to trial cannot be held more than the reasonable period of time necessary to determine whether there is a substantial probability that he will attain that capacity in the foreseeable future.[22]

This sounded like good news for accused persons. They would, at last, be given a chance to defend themselves in court. They would, finally, be considered innocent until proven guilty. If the prosecutor could not prove the criminal charges beyond a reasonable doubt, they would be free.

But in the very next sentence of its ruling, the Supreme Court took away from accused persons what it had seemed so close to giving them.

> If it is determined that this is not the case [their becoming competent in the foreseeable future], then the State must either institute the customary civil commitment proceedings that would be required to commit indefinitely any other citizen, or release the defendant.[23]

The Supreme Court thus shut the door on lifelong *criminal* confinement of persons never found guilty of any crime, but then opened wide the door to lifelong *civil* confinement for them. It virtually invited the states to continue warehousing defendants ruled incompetent for trial. The states have, indeed, found little difficulty in simply rewriting a few laws to comply with the label switching.[24]

California, for example, passed a law that simply defined *gravely disabled* as those inmates still considered incompetent for trial after three years' incarceration.[25] This means that even for those inmates who were released from the mental hospital, the state could maintain indefinite control through a conservatorship. Even though they might not be "gravely disabled" in any sense (unable to provide for food, clothing, or shelter as a result of mental disorder), nevertheless control could be maintained over their life, without offering them any of the constitutional due-process protections normally given to accused criminals. A lifetime of forced treatment with major tranquilizers would likely ensue.

A few years ago I was involved in a case that illustrates how convenient this label switching can be for the state. A man I'll call R. T. was accused in 1965 of assault, but was never brought to trial because psychiatrists examined him and reported to the court that he was incompetent to stand trial. In an uncontested hearing, the court accepted this finding and he was sent to a state hospital for the criminally insane.

Ten years later, R. T. was still incarcerated. For nine of those years, he was held as incompetent to stand trial, supposedly unable to understand charges and assist counsel. Then came the Supreme Court's *Jackson* decision.* Since R. T. had already been locked up for longer than "a reasonable period," the state would either have to place him on trial or (to quote the Court) "institute the customary civil commitment proceeding." Not surprisingly, the state chose civil commitment, since R. T.'s psychiatrists claimed he should continue to be held in a mental institution—and the state knew that a mental inmate of nine years' standing had little chance of convincing a judge or a jury to disagree with the doctors. This was much easier than having to prove R. T. was guilty of a crime.

When I was called by the public defender, R. T. had been on a conservatorship for one year. The hearing to renew this conservatorship, ordinarily a mere formality in which the judge accepts the doctor's recommendations, was this time going to be a full-blown jury trial. After ten years' incarceration, R. T. demanded that his public defender fight for his release from the hospital.

When I went to this hospital, I first reviewed R. T.'s medical records. I searched but could not find one word in ten years' worth of records to indicate that the psychiatrists had ever attempted to follow the law—that is, to evaluate R. T.'s competency for trial. Legally, indeed, R. T. was supposed to be denied trial only until the court found him able to understand the charges against him. Consistent with what researchers had shown to be a national pattern, the local court never commented on the hospital's failure to consider the question of competency. Instead, I found that psychiatrists kept R. T. in the hospital for nine years because they considered him "dangerous," even though during a decade of enforced institutionalization he had not been involved in a single violent incident.

_____
*Although the *Jackson* decision came three years before the events I am describing, it took that long for the case to have an impact on local practices.

R. T. had already served many more years in confinement than he would have served if he had been allowed to
stand trial and had been found guilty and sent to prison.
He was thus still locked up when the Supreme Court's
Jackson decision and a related California Supreme Court
ruling (*Davis*) came down.[26] Forced to respond to these
judicial rulings, the doctors had written to the local court:
"It is unlikely that he will ever regain his [competence for
trial] and be able to face his charges ... [A] report should be
made to court recommending that his charges be resolved
and that he be civilly committed to a state hospital."[27]
The psychiatrists were, in other words, following the letter
of the court's instructions: Continue the lockup, but just
do a little paper shuffling. Labels were switched and R. T.
was now called "gravely disabled."

In the year before my involvement, R. T. had obtained
a public defender, who was unable to convince the court
to release his client. Instead a county official was appointed
as conservator, and R. T. was ordered to "follow all medical recommendations. The current plan is continued hospitalization in an institution for the civilly committed."
The stage was set for him to spend the rest of his life in
a mental institution.

Yet one year later, R. T. was able to write the following letter to the public defender, even though he still carried a diagnosis of schizophrenia and had been continually
denied his right to stand trial on the grounds that he was
too confused to understand the criminal charges against him:

Dear Sir:

I would like you to file a petition in superior
court concerning conservatorship of R. T., conservatee.

I am requesting a hearing or jury trial before
the superior court instead of another year of conservatorship as petitioned by conservator, and discharge from present facility when present conservatorship terminates.

It was at this point, after nine years of penal confinement and one year of civil confinement, that the lawyer called me.

In talking with R. T., I was struck by the difference between the way he was described in his medical records and the manner in which he related to me. He was logical and coherent, interested most of all in getting out. Although he spoke in a soft voice, he seemed to show no hesitation in telling me about his background, the family problems prior to the criminal charges against him, and his ten years of confinement. As he continued his story, I began to gain some understanding of why the doctors would not release R. T.: He refused to talk to the doctors at the hospital. "If I get sore about being locked up," he explained, "they make me take drugs to calm me down." Somewhat later, he added, "I've had group therapy for ten years and I'll be damned if I'll do any more now."

R. T. had learned that if he expressed his frustration at being locked up for so many years, he was considered out of control and in need of more tranquilizers. Like virtually all inmates in mental institutions, he was kept on strong tranquilizers, and the dosage was increased whenever he showed any resentment, even verbally, toward what was being done to him. He had learned that it was wiser to keep his mouth shut about his feelings. But in the Catch-22 world of the mental institution, keeping his mouth shut was now hurting his chances of release. One of his doctors made the following note on his chart: "In order for him to be placed, he will have to talk to people . . . [He] shuts us out of his world." Another psychiatrist wrote along similar lines: "We have no idea what is going on in his mind . . . as long as he behaves in this manner it is difficult to consider placement in the community because I do not know what is going on in his mind."

As the date of his next conservatorship trial drew near, hospital psychiatrists decided to deny R. T. the right to be present in court. Since the chance to confront one's accusers is protected by the U.S. Constitution, this would be impossible in a criminal trial. But he was now a civilly committed "patient." Everything done now was "for" him rather than "to" him. Thus, when the decision to bar him from the conservatorship trial was made, his doctor declared that R. T. was "unable to attend the hearing" because "he will not talk to me or any other staff member; he does not socialize with anyone; he refuses to take part in any kind of activity; he paces all day long talking to himself."*

As it turned out, the trial never took place. The psychiatrists made a deal with R. T. in which they agreed to release him if he would agree to renewal of the conservatorship. He would be given a psychiatric parole, under the control of a conservator. This would mean, of course, that he would have to stay on powerful psychoactive drugs, live wherever the conservator told him to, and stay out of trouble. "Trouble" was not defined as breaking the law, but as anything that the conservator or the doctors considered bad for R. T.'s mental health. And of course they considered it bad for him to stop taking his tranquilizers. If he did this or anything else they disapproved of, he would be rehospitalized. After ten years of incarceration, awaiting a trial he was never granted, it seemed likely that he would remain under conservatorship for many years to come and perhaps for the rest of his life.

The Man Who Wasn't There

Before concluding this chapter, let me offer one more illustration to show how a psychiatric pronouncement of incompetence for trial may be used as a tactic by the

---

*Pacing, secondary to a profound sense of restlessness, is a common side effect of the major tranquilizers. Trying to combat this discomfort, persons receiving these drugs keep on the move. The syndrome is called akathisia.

defense lawyer in preparing for an insanity defense.[28] In Hawaii a Marine on several occasions in 1978 raped pre-teen-age girls and forced them to perform fellatio on him. Particularly noteworthy, in light of what would later be said about his being unfit for trial, was the cunning he used in luring his victims. On a typical occasion he spotted his victim walking on a quiet road. He jogged past her, around a curve, and then jumped into a construction ditch by the side of the road. As she walked past, he yelled for help, saying he had tripped and fallen and hurt his leg. He asked her to help him get out. When she tried to help, he pulled her down and sexually assaulted her. On another occasion he spotted a girl on a bicycle and told her someone had been hurt. Would she please come and help carry the injured person out of the woods? Anxious to help, the girl followed him to an isolated spot, only to become his next victim.

When this man was finally caught, his lawyer decided to use a psychiatric defense. The factual evidence against him was overwhelming. After several psychiatrists examined him but could find no signs of mental disorder, the lawyer finally found a psychologist from California who claimed the defendant was a multiple personality. A "secondary ego state" had taken over and committed the rapes. This ultimately became the grounds for a plea of not guilty by reason of insanity, but even before this plea was entered, the defense lawyers argued the man should be sent to a hospital as unfit to stand trial.

The reason? The "other" personality, the guilty one, could not be present at the trial, since he was buried somewhere in the unconscious mind of the accused. The man sitting in court should be sent to a mental hospital where the two personalities could be "fused into one." Then the trial could proceed. Even though neither the defense lawyers nor the psychiatrists claimed the defendant was confused about what was taking place, the judge granted this request. The accused was found unfit for trial.

For more than a year, at great expense to the taxpayers of Hawaii, this man's trial was delayed while psychiatrists set about "fusing two personalities." Finally the psychiatrists claimed he was ready for trial. The court now heard the plea: not guilty by reason of insanity. The same psychiatrists testified that the criminally responsible party, the "other" personality, had disappeared as a result of treatment. The one sitting in court should be excused.

Solely on the basis of psychiatric testimony (a full trial was never held), the defendant was pronounced legally insane and returned to the mental institution. But unlike R.T., who was warehoused years longer than if he had been found guilty and sent to prison, this man will almost certainly be released years sooner than if he had been found guilty. Even as he was pronounced legally insane, the psychiatrists were testifying that he was no longer dangerous because they had succeeded in blending his evil personality into his good personality.

Reforms

When the Supreme Court handed down its ruling in the *Jackson* case, in 1972, most experts believed that the injustices surrounding determinations of incompetence to stand trial would become a thing of the past. That did not happen. Rather, the high court invited the states to expand the powers of the mental health system while moving to reduce the powers of the criminal justice system. This was an inadequate solution.

The Court failed to probe deeply enough, never asking the fundamental questions, such as whether psychiatric opinions are necessary in determining whether a person understands the charges and can rationally assist a lawyer. The Court also failed to seriously question whether a finding of incompetence for trial was really intended to help the accused person.

Our courts will continue to make convenient use of incompetence-for-trial rulings until we confront these issues more directly. The proper beginning of honest reform, not mere label switching, is a recognition that psychiatrists cannot help. The psychiatrist's report only makes it easier for the judge, the prosecutor, or the defense lawyer to use the hearings for hidden purposes.

With the removal of the psychiatrists, we could seek to accomplish three objectives. First, those few defendants unable to understand the charges or rationally assist counsel would have a chance to get help before a trial, but would also be protected from unwanted and punishing involuntary psychiatric treatment. Second, defendants' rights to a speedy trial would be protected. Third, society's right to a speedy trial would be protected, and prosecutors would have a fair chance to prove guilt. Our current policies accomplish none of these objectives. The following procedures would accomplish all of them.

First, *only the defense lawyer, never the judge or the prosecutor, may request a competency hearing.* If competency hearings are truly aimed at protecting the defendant from an unfair trial, why should prosecutors and judges be allowed to raise this issue? They represent the state, not the defendant, and can be easily tempted by their positions to seek a finding of incompetence for reasons having nothing to do with the defendant's welfare.

Second, *once the defense lawyer raises the issue, a competency hearing should take place, and no psychiatric examinations or testimony would be permitted.* Instead, the defense would present witnesses who would testify about what they have observed of the defendant's behavior since the arrest. The defendant's state of mind would be evaluated by the judge or jury, through his or her testimony.* The defense attorney could also be questioned by the judge.

---

*Defendants may not be forced to testify in a criminal trial, but they are required to be examined by a psychiatrist once the question of competence is raised. Requiring their testimony at a competency hearing would thus not deny them any constitutional rights.

The prosecutor may, of course, call adverse witnesses or be content to cross-examine the defendant's witnesses. All defendants would be presumed competent unless a preponderance of the evidence points to incompetence. Those found competent would proceed to trial. Those found incompetent would proceed to step three, below. If the prosecutor should decide to accept the defendant's claim that he or she is incompetent to stand trial, no hearing would occur; rather the judge would proceed to step three, below.

Third, *a grace period for those held to be incompetent would be granted, whereby trial would be delayed for a period not to exceed six months.* Based on the nature of the alleged crime and related facts, the judge would decide whether the defendant would remain in confinement during this grace period or be released. If the accused is to be confined, the defendant may request that the pretrial period be spent in a locked mental facility rather than in a jail. The judge may grant this request, but may not *order* the defendant to be involuntarily confined in a mental facility. Once in a mental facility, moreover, the defendant would be free to accept or reject any suggested treatment.

If the defendant is released pending trial, he or she would be free to seek psychiatric services, but would be under no obligation to do so. Since trial would in any case proceed within six months, the untreated accused could not elude criminal prosecution indefinitely; society thus would not need to insist that treatment be given. The defendant, moreover, may request that the trial begin at any time prior to the six-month deadline, but may not delay the trial beyond this deadline.

This three-step plan offers distinct advantages to the defense, to the prosecution, and to society. Defendants would be protected from the punishment of involuntary psychiatric treatments. Whatever treatment they received, if any, would be legitimate (voluntary) treatment instead of quasi-criminal punishment. Defendants would also be

protected from the lengthy mental hospitalization that
denies them the right to a speedy trial.

The prosecutor, knowing that a trial will not be delayed longer than six months, need not worry about losing
witnesses or having their memories fade. Society, finally,
would receive two main benefits. First, society's wish to
prosecute those accused of crime and punish those found
guilty would be reflected in the procedure dictating a
mandatory trial after six months. Second, society's wish to
be fair to mentally disordered persons would be reflected
both in the grace period and in the abandonment of the
practice of forcing any accused person to accept psychiatric treatments. Because the trial would proceed within
six months, regardless of the defendant's mental state, no
official in any capacity could operate under the assumption that the untreated person would forever escape criminal prosecution. Society would instead be saying to the
incompetent defendant, "We will leave you alone to seek
help in your own way, but only for six months."

Supporters of our current methods might immediately
argue that even after six months it would still be unfair
to place on trial the person who continues to be seriously
disturbed and unable to understand the charges. To those
who hold this view I assert that of the two possibilities—
a criminal trial or a civil commitment proceeding—the
criminal trial is far more fair and far more capable of
allowing the defendant to receive justice. A civil commitment proceeding is far more risky than is a criminal trial,
for in a civil commitment trial there are far fewer legal
protections than in a criminal trial. In a civil commitment
trial, proof of accusations need only be shown by a "preponderance of evidence." In a criminal trial, on the other
hand, the state is required to prove its claims "beyond a
reasonable doubt." In a civil commitment trial, a judge
or jury may be tempted to commit the person to an institution, because this is considered "helpful." In a criminal
trial, the result of a guilty verdict is recognized as punish-

ment, so the judge or jury will be more concerned about the facts of the case. In a civil commitment trial, confinement, perhaps for life, is considered therapeutic. So much for being "fair" to the mentally disordered by sparing them a criminal trial. If a grossly disordered person faces possible incarceration following a criminal act, he or she deserves the full constitutional protections that only a criminal trial provides.

A Ban on Psychiatric Testimony

I cannot discuss in this book each of the many other types of hearings or trials in which psychiatric testimony is utilized. Decisions about drug addiction, guardianship, marriage, divorce, child custody, adoption, contracts, wills, disability payments, personal injury claims, consent for medical treatment, job hiring and firing, government security clearances, detection of lying, military discharges, are all situations in which we turn to the psychiatrist for "expert" advice. Although I have not been able to discuss each one, I am ready to make the following blanket recommendation: *In any of these cases, psychiatric opinions should neither be solicited nor permitted.* In each case, a particular question needs answering. Often the dilemmas are indeed difficult. But in no case does the psychiatrist (or psychologist) have anything truly "expert" or "special" to offer. Instead, the judge, jury, or hearing officer should hear the testimony of those persons with first-hand information. From this information will emerge the basis for a decision on the questions before the court.

Why is this alternative preferable to our currently strong reliance on psychiatric examinations? Because judges and juries would have to restrict themselves to the concrete testimony of lay witnesses, and would not be left confused by "expert" psychiatric speculations. The decision-making process would only be improved by the recognition that in cases involving possible emotional injury from someone's negligent behavior, or in cases involving issues of mental capacity and intent, we have no need to call in the experts, because there are no experts.

Some may think I am presumptuous in urging that in every one of these areas psychiatrists be excluded. But I believe it is psychiatry and our traditional reliance on psychiatry that are presumptuous. We presume that psychiatry can do more than it can. The burden of proof should now fall, I believe, on those who argue that we should *continue* our courtroom addiction to psychiatry.

CHAPTER 6

A MATTER OF CONSENT
Lessons from Psychiatry's Past

Among doctors, only psychiatrists may impose treatment on unwilling patients. The rationale for this appears to be sound: Mental illness impairs rational choice, whereas medical illness does not. I want to question this reasoning, for my experience as a psychiatrist leads me to believe that mental patients should also have the power of consent. Why? Because denial of the right to consent makes mental patients into second-class citizens and leaves them more vulnerable to harm, not less.

Let us look briefly at the track record compiled by psychiatry, focusing on the result of giving psychiatrists the legal authority to impose treatment. Because of this authority, time and again the most respected leaders of psychiatry, as well as their lesser-known colleagues, have imposed treatments that patients resisted and that were later regretted by all. These lessons from the past may be useful should we decide to question the authority of today's psychiatrist to have the final say.

"The Father of American Psychiatry"

During whatever period in time one chooses to examine, one finds that an amazing variety of manipulations of the mind and body have been foisted on mental patients by their doctors. One of the most inventive among these was Benjamin Rush, a signer of the Declaration of Independence and from 1783 to 1813 director of the mental ward

111

at the Pennsylvania Hospital. Rush is considered "the father of American psychiatry," and his likeness appears on the seal of the American Psychiatric Association. Even more than most doctors of his day, Rush was an enthusiastic practitioner of bleeding, eventually earning the title the "lancet loving physician of Philadelphia."[1] Sometimes Rush removed as much as half of the patient's total blood volume. He theorized that madness was caused by too much blood in the brain, and claimed that his theory was proved by autopsy findings of "preternatural hardness" of the brain.[2]

There is no question that massive bleeding changed Rush's patients, at least for a while. Although he described the change as a cure, we now know he was merely putting the patient into vascular shock. Extreme blood loss leads to a drop in blood pressure. With inadequate circulation of blood to the brain, the person becomes confused and apathetic. All persons, not just those considered mad, will respond in this way. In simple terms, Rush was altering the patient's mental state by bleeding, and then convincing himself that the change was a cure and was proof that a brain disorder had responded to treatment. Both ideas are now easily recognized as foolish.

Rush was also proud of his "tranquilizer." Unlike today's tranquilizers, Rush's invention was a specially designed chair that held the patient's body completely immobilized. What was the purpose of total restraint? Bleeding and intestinal purging could be performed despite the protests of the patient. Rush touted the tranquilizer's advantages over the straitjacket (camisole). Whereas the older device "renders it impracticable to bleed them," his new chair allowed the doctor to "retain all the benefits of coercion." These benefits included the fact that he could "open a vein without relieving any other part of the body from its confinement," and he could administer intestinal purges "without subjecting the patient to the necessity of being moved from his chair or exposing him afterwards to the fetor of his excretions or to their contact with his body."[3]

Cutting the Personality to Measure

If Benjamin Rush could justify bleeding to correct an imaginary excess of blood in the brain, perhaps it is not too surprising that in our own times doctors could rationalize the slicing of millions of nerve cells in a patient's brain. Madness was no longer the result of excess blood; instead, brain circuits were "reverberating" and acting in other strange ways. The patient would be better off without unruly brain tissue.

Walter Freeman, a neurologist who practiced brain surgery on mental patients, was the most noted proponent and popularizer of frontal lobotomy.[4] Fifty thousand frontal lobotomies were performed in America, mostly during the 1940s and 1950s, and Freeman performed about four thousand of them.[5] His work was widely praised in the popular press as a way to "cut the personality to measure, sounding a note of hope for those who are afflicted with insanity."[6] Freeman's activities were also widely discussed by psychiatrists. Not all of them liked what he was doing, but Freeman certainly held positions indicating that his activities were considered praiseworthy. From 1927 to 1954 he was a faculty member at the George Washington University Hospital and from 1934 to 1946 he was the secretary of the American Board of Psychiatry and Neurology. He lectured widely and wrote in great detail about his work, particularly in his book *Psychosurgery*, co-authored with neurosurgeon James Watts. The book first appeared in 1942; a revised edition was published in 1950.[7]

What happened during these lobotomies? Here is how a medical student described what she saw. The year was 1949.

My medical school class was invited to see a demonstration of such a transorbital lobotomy, one of several types of lobotomies. The neurosurgeon, on the staff of a university medical school, stood before the class strutting in a sedate, self-important manner. I remember how good looking and smooth he appeared, a typical Hollywood symbol of the handsome doctor whose patients go ga-ga over him . . . and how entirely devoid of character he was. He was meticulously groomed, hair perfectly in place, skin very white and smooth-shaven—a perfect, successful representative of White Anglo-Saxon America. He wore a suit and tie and looked as if he were addressing a business-men's luncheon meeting of the Kiwanis Club. After some introductory remarks he opened the door and the nurse and orderly pushed a stretcher into the room. Walking in with them was an attractive young black man, eighteen years old, looking frightened and bewildered. The neurosurgeon paid no attention to him but continued discussing with us how the operation would be conducted, and he seemed proud of the fact that they didn't even need anesthesia for the operation—that knocking the patient out with "a couple of electric shock treatments" would be adequate anesthetization. . .

The young black man in wrinkled hospital garb stood cowering in the corner in sharp contrast with the urbane, smooth, self-possessed polished physician. Finally the doctor turned to the patient, mentioned his diagnosis . . . Schizophrenic Reaction . . . and that he was a recent hospital admission . . . and told him to get up on the stretcher. The young man backed up, his shoulders hunched like a scared cat being attacked by a growling bulldog, his eyes darting this way and that in a futile attempt to seek some way of escape from the inevitable. The nurse and orderly then held his arms, brought him to the stretcher, and somehow managed to get him to lie down on it, shackling his wrists and ankles. The doctor applied the electrodes to the young man's temples, the current was turned on, and the young man's body jerked convulsively for several seconds. The doctor said smoothly, as though nothing had happened, that he thought he'd give another dose of electric current to be sure he's knocked out completely. Again the current was turned on, again the captured victim was convulsively responding with his entire body to the electricity searing his brain cells.

. . . The patient was, after the second electric shock, completely limp and "anesthetized." I have never, neither before nor since that incident, heard of using electricity for anesthesia! The surgeon then took an instrument *from his pocket* in a pointedly and overly nonchalant manner and showed the ice-pick-like tool to the class. He then lifted one eyelid of the patient's and stuck the pick up—he made a point of showing that he was having some trouble getting the pick through the skull and into the brain at the first try and he grimaced at the class and said something about the "thickness of the boy's skull." A few of the more obvious racists in the class gave him his anticipated reply by snickering—some of the students, already uncomfortable, had their discomfort increased at this remark. After the pick had penetrated the skull, he flicked his wrist back and forth with the pick slashing into the brain substance, severing forever, in an instant, those connections that nature had labored to achieve over millions of years.

I was not the only one who gasped at the outrage I had just witnessed. One girl, Dottie, her head probably full of the sterile operative techniques

with sterilization of instruments we'd been taught
to observe prior to and during the operation, raised
her hand and asked about using an unsterilized
instrument, to which the surgeon retorted with a
pretty-boy smile: "Well, I didn't wipe it on my
bootstrap."[8]

Shock Treatment: As Damaging as Ever

Shock treatment started in 1933, with insulin being used
to drop the patient's blood sugar low enough to cause a
coma and sometimes a convulsion.[9] This was the idea of
Manfred Sakel, who had been treating his private patients
at the Lichterfelder sanitarium, near Berlin, in this manner
for several years. Sakel's reasoning was the following:

My supposition was that some noxious agent weak-
ened the resilience and the metabolism of the nerve
cells . . . a reduction in the energy spending of the
cell, that is in invoking a minor or greater hiberna-
tion in it, by blocking the cell off with insulin will
force it to conserve functional energy and store it
to be available for the re-enforcement of the cell.[10]

In just a few years after Sakel published his new method
insulin shock treatment was being used on thousands of
the world's mental patients. Today it is rarely used.

Laszlo von Meduna had a different theory, one he
developed during the early 1930s while working at the
Interacademic Brain Research Institute in Budapest.
Meduna based his new "Metrazol shock" on the idea,
now completely discredited, that epileptics almost never
become schizophrenic and schizophrenics almost never
become epileptic. If epilepsy somehow prevented schizophrenia, he reasoned, why not cause the schizophrenic to
become epileptic (at least temporarily) by causing him or
her to convulse?[11] Perhaps these convulsions would make
the schizophrenia go away.

Meduna used a chemical (Metrazol*), rather than the hormone insulin, to produce the convulsions. Like insulin, Metrazol was given by intravenous injection. Before the patient started to convulse, he or she experienced a horrible period of panic and impending doom, lasting up to a minute. It was not a popular treatment.

Ugo Cerletti, professor of neuropsychiatry at the University of Rome, conceived the method by which shock treatment is given today—electric shock. Cerletti accepted the idea that convulsions were good for schizophrenics, and in 1938 started using electric shock to produce the convulsions.[12] Electric shock treatment quickly replaced insulin and Metrazol as the favorite form of shock treatment, and became the most effective method of controlling troublesome asylum inmates.

Today between one hundred thousand and two hundred thousand Americans receive electroconvulsive treatment (ECT) each year.[13] About 120 volts, the amount in ordinary house current, is applied to the brain for about a half-second. A course of treatment usually lasts two to three weeks, with shocks given perhaps ten to fifteen times. Some doctors give several shocks at a time, one right after the other. Many patients have received over the years several courses of treatment, and some patients are even "maintained" on shock treatments indefinitely. Many people believe that shock therapy is no longer dangerous. This is because psychiatry proudly proclaims that shock treatment today is administered differently from earlier practices.

I first witnessed shock treatment in 1963, when I visited the Illinois State Hospital at Manteno with three other University of Chicago medical students. After being shown around several of the wards, we were taken to observe patients receive "shock." Expecting to enter a treatment room with two or three patients waiting outside, we

---

*Metrazol is the trade name for Pentylenetetrazol.

instead found ourselves inside a cavernous ward. About two dozen patients, lying on their backs and strapped to treatment tables, were lined up from one end of the room to the other. Most were women.

The treating psychiatrist greeted us and got to work. I had the impression, by the way the doctor readied her equipment, that administering shock treatment was routine. As the other patients watched, she rubbed conducting paste on the temples of the first patient, a woman who appeared to be in her forties. She passively accepted the rubber mouthpiece placed in her mouth, as though she had done this many times. We were told the mouthpiece was to prevent cuts during the seizure.

The doctor pressed a button on the small box she had been adjusting and the convulsion began. The woman went rigid and then began to convulse rhythmically. Her face became a ghastly blue as her convulsing muscles prevented her from breathing. It seemed like a long time before she started to breathe again, but it was probably only a few seconds. She made grunting and snorting sounds, as saliva, mixed with a little blood, frothed at the corners of her mouth. Once it was clear that she would continue to breathe, perhaps thirty seconds to a minute after the shock had been given, the doctor went to the next patient. Most of the patients seemed prepared to accept the treatment without complaint, and a few told the doctor they were doing better and could skip a treatment today. Such pleas went unheeded.

We watched two or three more treatments, as the doctor made her way down the line of carts. We were told this was a typical day: Shock was given between ten and eleven o'clock each morning. We then moved on to other sights and sounds of the hospital.

Today fewer patients are given ECT. The practice is no longer common in state mental hospitals, but is still used widely in private mental hospitals. Psychiatrists who currently administer shock therapy claim it is a lifesaving treatment for those who are severely depressed and possibly suicidal. Furthermore, they insist that ECT no longer deserves its ugly reputation, because there have been several new medical developments in how the treatment is administered.

Today's patient is first injected with a barbiturate; thus the person is unconscious before the electric shock is administered. Second, he or (usually) she is given a nerve-blocking agent (succinylcholine), which paralyzes the muscles of the body. As a result, the outward muscular convulsion is greatly reduced. In the past, patients sometimes suffered bone fractures or dislocations from muscular convulsions. Third, oxygen is given to the patient, to compensate for the patient's inability to breathe; thus the patient does not become cyanotic (blue).

Proponents of ECT claim these developments make shock treatment safe and effective. Psychiatrist Stuart Yudofsky of the New York State Psychiatric Institute, for example, has said, "The only way you physically know a seizure is taking place is that sometimes you see a finger wiggling slightly."[14]

What Yudofsky is really saying, I believe, is that *shock treatment is now easier for the psychiatrist to watch.* In truth the electricity coursing through the brain is no less damaging now than it was forty years ago.[15] In fact, the sedating drugs now given prior to the shock require the doctor to use somewhat higher doses of electricity, since it takes more current to produce a brain seizure.[16]

The electric current injures the brain's tissue, causing mental confusion. The medical developments described above, in other words, have done nothing to change how shock treatment "works": the patient is so dazed and confused that he or she forgets many important things. For a few weeks, emotional problems are driven from the mind, but they are not solved or alleviated in any way. Neurologist Sidney Sament has described what happens.

I have seen many patients after ECT, and I have no doubt that ECT produces effects identical to those of a head injury. After multiple sessions of ECT, a patient has symptoms identical to those of a retired, punch-drunk boxer. After one session of ECT the symptoms are the same as those of a concussion (including retrograde and anterograde amnesia). After a few sessions of ECT the symptoms are those of moderate cerebral contusion, and further enthusiastic use of ECT may result in the patient functioning at a subhuman level. Electroconvulsive therapy in effect may be defined as a controlled type of brain damage produced by electrical means. No doubt some psychiatric symptoms are eliminated . . . but this is at the expense of the brain damage, which may have varying effects on patients' lives, depending on their age, personality and the number of ECT treatments. In all cases the ECT "response" is due to the concussion-type, or more serious, effects of ECT. The patient "forgets" his symptoms because the brain damage destroys memory traces in the brain, and the patient has to pay for this by a reduction in mental capacity of varying degree . . . a patient "responding" to ECT and even becoming asymptomatic and "easier to manage" is not necessarily healthy or cured but may be functioning at a low mental level, and his potential for full human function may be seriously impaired.[17]

The causes of the patient's depression—marital or interpersonal stress, financial pressures, problems of aging—are untouched by ECT. The patient's *concern* over these problems is temporarily blotted out, but soon (usually after a few weeks or a month) the brain recovers enough for the person to remember his or her problems. Now the patient has an additional reason to feel low: Memory for past events and ability to retain new information are impaired. The brain injury leaves residual damage that may be permanent.

There is disagreement among researchers on the likelihood of permanent damage.[18] This is because the "tests" used in psychiatry and psychology are strictly subjective and open to interpretation. Proponents of ECT readily admit the treatment's immediate impact on memory and learning but deny that this is long lasting. They say that the common complaints of ECT recipients, even those made years later, are a result of their mental disorders, not the result of treatment.[19]

I am unable to dismiss these complaints so easily, since many ECT recipients describe what clinical medicine teaches us to expect from a brain injury. Brain injuries, particularly those involving the areas that ECT selects (temporal lobes and the underlying structures), may cause permanent memory loss for events in the past (retrograde amnesia). Memory of the months immediately before and after the injury is especially vulnerable. Brain injuries may also cause permanent deficiencies in retention of new information (anterograde amnesia). It is this learning disability that is particularly upsetting for recipients. I have talked with many ECT recipients: Some of them have no complaints of permanent deficiencies, but most do.

If psychiatrists who use ECT deny the possibility of permanent injury, among themselves and to the public, they are hardly likely to mention the possibility to patients asked to consent to the treatment. Instead, patients are told that confusion and memory impairment last just a few weeks. Merely this lack of accurate information on which the patient may decide whether the risks of treatment are worth the potential benefits makes suspect the apparent consent of most ECT recipients. Equally important is the legal and ethical requirement that the consent be truly free. But is free consent possible on a psychiatric ward, where patients (even those who appear to be voluntary) may not leave unless the psychiatrist agrees? True voluntary status is rather uncommon on a mental ward.[20] Finally, one last factor makes these dilemmas of consent even more troublesome. Once the patient has received the first or second of the ten or twelve treatments planned, he or she is so confused that any resistance to the treatment has been wiped out. Even if the patient had the physical capacity to fight back, he or she has lost the desire to do so.

Shock treatment is now enjoying a renaissance because of psychiatry's strong promotion of medical rather than psychological treatment methods. Whereas twenty years ago it was considered an embarrassment to psychiatry, ECT is once again being vigorously promoted. And like every other instance, past and present, in which physical intrusion becomes a "treatment" simply by official pronouncement, ECT is now said to correct brain abnormality. Some have likened it to "recharging our batteries."[21] Others, hoping to sound more scientific, have said it "stimulates the deeper survival centers of the brain."[22]

Shock treatment thus follows in the path of earlier treatments, like bleeding or lobotomy, now discarded by psychiatry. But there is no sign yet that ECT is about to be relegated to the past. A treatment favored by psychiatry will be used regardless of the cost to the patient and regardless of the patient's wishes.

Operation Mind Control: Missing the Point

When clear-cut examples of mental patient abuse come to light, we often overlook the most basic reason: the patient's powerlessness to refuse an unwanted treatment. A dramatic example was the 1975 disclosure that the CIA and the army, employing some of psychiatry's most established figures, had for twenty-five years been conducting "mind control" experiments.[23] The Rockefeller Commission study of the CIA was the beginning of these disclosures.

When the government's mind control experiments came to light, critics challenged both the intelligence agencies and cooperating doctors, but overlooked the most crucial factor of all. They overlooked the fact that these crude experiments were routinely performed on powerless mental patients without any help from the CIA or the army. Critics accused the doctors more for working for the government than for the tortures they were perpetrating on mental patients. To illustrate, let us consider one of the experiments performed for the Army Chemical Corps.

Harold Blauer died the day before he was scheduled to be discharged from the New York State Psychiatric Institute. His family was told he had suffered an unexpected reaction to one of his treatments. In fact, a team of doctors was conducting secret experiments for the Army Chemical Corps, in which patients were injected with mescaline and other psychoactive drugs. The army was trying to develop drugs that would control the mind.

Despite Blauer's great discomfort and growing resistance, he was subjected to higher and higher dosage levels with each succeeding injection. On January 8, 1953, less than one month after the first injection, the doctors gave him a dose sixteen times greater than the original one. Moments later he died. Immediately, the army and the Justice Department made every effort to cover up the cause of death. Even the New York deputy chief medical examiner cooperated by reporting that Blauer had died from aggravation of a "previously undetected heart problem."[24] The chief investigator was Paul Hoch, head of the Department of Experimental Psychiatry at the institute. He later became New York State commissioner of mental hygiene, and was a major figure in psychiatry.

Experimentation with psychiatric patients did not begin with the CIA and army funding. It was already being performed on inmates of mental asylums. Doctors like Hoch had already published work of this type in psychiatry's leading journals, to the applause of their fellow psychiatrists. This is how the CIA and the army knew which doctors to approach for experiments that might accomplish intelligence or military objectives.

In the 1950s and 1960s, drugs like LSD and mescaline were popular among experimenters. Many believed that these drugs could induce a "model psychosis," by which psychiatry could gain new insights into mental disorder. In the February 1951 issue of the *American Journal of Psychiatry*, Hoch and his colleagues described the effects of mescaline injection: restlessness, tremor, dilated pupils, psychosis, anxiety, and sometimes panic.[25] Of the three cases they discussed, two were subjected to lobotomy and then reinjected with mescaline. In some cases, shock treatment was given after the mescaline injections, in an attempt to blot out the fear and panic produced by the drugs. If that didn't work, the subject was given still other drugs. In a dozen papers, published in the posthumous collection aptly entitled *The Complete Psychiatrist*, Hoch further discussed his experimental research.[26] Hoch was eulogized not only by psychiatry's most respected figures but also by New York governors Nelson Rockefeller and Averell Harriman.

He was praised as well by the very influential psychiatrist D. Ewen Cameron. Like Hoch, Cameron conducted secret experiments for government intelligence agencies; like Hoch, Cameron died before his undercover work became known to the general public in 1975; like Hoch, Cameron was a major figure in psychiatry (president of the American Psychiatric Association in 1953, the first president of the World Psychiatric Association, and the director of McGill University's prestigious Allen Memorial Institute). And finally, like Hoch, Cameron also did the very same things out in the open, to professional acclaim, when secret government money was not involved.

Although Cameron liberally administered a wide variety of drugs, his notoriety now comes from his application of massive doses of electroshock, something he called depatterning.[27] By shocking patients many times a day, Cameron rendered them so stuporous that they were unable to eat, dress, or control their urine and bowels, and had no memory and little intellect. Cameron justified this by claiming that the subjects were "completely free from all emotional disturbance, save for a customary mild euphoria."

Cameron attracted the attention of the CIA primarily because he frankly admitted that memory loss was not a "side effect" of shock treatment but rather the desired and directly "therapeutic" effect. Memory loss, he wrote, was "an essential part of the recovery process." He theorized that as memory improved after the shocks were stopped, only normal thoughts would return while the "diseased" thinking would be left behind forever. Even though Cameron had absolutely no evidence to support this claim, the CIA was interested in him because it wanted to find a way to erase the memories of its own agents who upon retirement might leak secret information. As minutes of a CIA conference noted, "Some of the individuals in the Agency had to know tremendous amounts of information and if a way could be found to produce amnesia . . . after the individual left the Agency, it would be a remarkable thing.[28]

Both Hoch and Cameron, as well as countless others, illustrate the danger confronting patients when we deny them the right of informed and free consent to psychiatric treatment. By denying mental patients the power of consent our society puts them in great danger. Once denied the final say, mental patients become vulnerable to whatever manipulations psychiatrists decide to call treatment. Many of these so-called treatments have been crude experiments and sometimes they were no less than torture.[29]

What lesson may be drawn from this history? Our society has given psychiatry the power over treatment in the belief that mental patients are not able to handle the decisions, but psychiatrists have not demonstrated the ability to make wise decisions about treatment. I *submit that the primary lesson of psychiatry's past is that mental patients are better qualified to decide to accept or reject a treatment than are psychiatrists.*

Psychiatry's favored treatment today is psychoactive drugs. But psychiatry's drug revolution is more of a retreat than a revolution, and only confirms the lessons from psychiatry's past.

CHAPTER 7

PSYCHIATRY'S NEW DRUGS
Revolution or Retreat?

In our time drugs are being hailed as the best treatment for major mental disorders. They are nothing less than revolutionary, modern psychiatry tells us, because they treat chemically what is fundamentally a biochemical disorder. Psychiatry has discovered that serious mental problems are the result of faulty brain chemistry.[1]

One way psychiatry supports its claims is to point to an indisputable statistic: Today's mental hospitals house only one-half to one-third as many patients as they did a mere twenty-five years ago.[2] The reason for this dramatic change, psychiatry says, is drugs; because "antipsychotic" medications treat the biochemical disorder that causes schizophrenia, many chronic patients can be discharged from the hospital setting and returned to their communities.[3] The decline in the number of patients in mental institutions is certainly not to be challenged, but the explanation for the wave of discharges during the 1950s and 1960s deserves closer consideration.

Dollars and Cents

Mental hospitals in the United States now hold fewer patients, not primarily because of drugs, but mainly for economic reasons. It simply became too expensive to house a large number of patients in state mental hospitals.[4] In the 1950s, private, state, and veterans hospitals were bulging with nearly a million patients. Huge numbers of patients were housed in state mental institutions simply because they had no money to pay for needed services in the community. The state hospital served quite simply as a dumping ground. Then, in the late 1950s and 1960s, social and fiscal policy changes were enacted in response to the high cost of running large institutions. First, Social Security laws were amended to provide benefits to discharged patients. The vast number of elderly citizens who had been placed in a state asylum by their families were now able to pay for nursing homes. Many had never been "mentally ill" in the first place; rather they were senile, helpless, and forgotten. Second, local governments were given federal money to treat patients in the community instead of in the state hospital. And in 1963 mental patients could for the first time receive disability income, so that those unable to work were not completely penniless. Mental hospitals were then less needed to function as poorhouses. Since the advent of welfare payments, the states have been particularly tempted to release mental patients because the money for community support is supplied by the federal government, whereas state mental hospital costs are paid by the state.[5]

Joseph O'Connor was assistant commissioner of mental health for the city of New York in 1974 and 1975 and saw the economic forces at work. His job was to keep the mental health budget within acceptable limits, and through his position he saw clearly why patients were released from state mental hospitals and what role drugs played. During a recent interview he recalled those years. "The state mental health population," he began,

> had been around 75,000 patients and the majority came from the big cities, particularly New York City, because of the socioeconomic conditions of the city and its large minority and poverty populations. They were the majority of the tenants in the state institutions.

As a result of the Civil Rights Act of 1964, people incarcerated in state mental institutions that had physical ailments were to be released or sent to a medical institution. Things like arteriosclerosis [senility]. We had lumped everybody in the state institutions. So, Governor Carey and his state mental health commissioner decided this was a perfect time to open the doors of the institutions and say they shouldn't be here. We'd save the state a lot of money because at that time the state was paying 75 percent of the dollars and the federal government was paying 25 percent.

"Are you saying," I asked, "that most of those people released were senile old people?"
"The majority." he answered.

The directors of state mental institutions were under great pressure to cut their budgets and the best way to do that was to cut the population. Our state hospital population shrank to around 30,000 and most of those people that were let go came back to the cities. They became the residents of the SRO—single room occupancy—hotels, so then the city was responsible, not the state. The state now only had to pay 25 percent—not 75 percent— while the city paid 50 percent and the federal government 25 percent. So this became a big fiscal problem for the city of New York.

"What about medications?" I asked. "Was that important in the shift?" His reply challenges the statements of psychiatrists:

This whole aspect had nothing at all to do with medicine. It was a fiscal situation. I'm just a layman, of course, but as far as I could see it had nothing to do with that. The only thing I could see the drugs did was to sedate the people and get 'em dreary and droopy. They certainly couldn't function in a big city community. The whole thing was born not out of design but of necessity—when the state mental health department realized that they found a new trick that could save a lot of money by decertifying everybody.[6]

If mental patients were moved from large state institutions to community placements as a result of economic considerations rather than drugs, this does not imply that this shift was not necessary. Despite the overwhelming adjustment problems faced by many discharged patients and the fact that most of them have been badly neglected in the community, deinstitutionalization is a necessary first step toward enlightened policies on mental deviance.

When it is recognized that financial considerations were the major reason for the huge wave of mental hospital discharges, then the role of drugs is seen in a different light. Medication undoubtedly facilitated many discharges, by dulling patients and making them more compliant, but medication only served to assist—it did not make possible— patient release. Lowered mental hospital populations thus prove nothing about the nature of mental disorders.

The economic basis of deinstitutionalization also does not imply that psychiatric medications are never of help. Some patients seem to benefit from them and take them willingly because they feel the calming effect is worth a degree of diminished alertness. But it makes a difference whether a patient takes medication because he or she finds it helpful or because the patient believes the doctor has discovered a brain abnormality that can be treated with drugs. Millions of patients are now told by their doctors to stay on psychoactive medications for years or even a lifetime. Psychiatry now teaches that disordered brain metabolism is the problem and long-term medication is the answer.

We must ask why psychiatry is so anxious to promote its theories about a chemical basis of schizophrenia or depression, as if such theories were proven medical fact. To answer this question we need to examine the relationship between psychiatry and the manufacturers of mind-altering drugs.

Pills and Profits

Drug company profits had much to do with promoting the idea that deinstitutionalization of mental patients resulted primarily from revolutionary new drugs. Although chlorpromazine, for example, had been subjected to few studies when it was first marketed in mid-1954, by the end of the year it was being given to an estimated two million mental patients in the United States alone. This one drug played a significant role in the increase in net sales of the Smith, Kline and French firm from $53 million in 1953 to $347 million in 1970.[7] Profits have continued to be enormous, making the pharmaceutical industry a leading profit maker among the world's manufacturing industries.[8]

At a recent convention of the American Psychiatric Association, the intimate tie between psychiatry and the pharmaceutical business was very much in evidence, from the cocktail parties hosted by drug companies to the mass dissemination of free literature praising each company's products. Pamphlets touted a "novel antidepressant" drug, a new drug for senility, and another for hyperactive children. Another pamphlet hailed a liquid tranquilizer that could be secretly introduced into a stubborn patient's food.[9] While psychiatrists and physicians in general claim they do not take drug company literature seriously, studies of the drug-prescribing habits of doctors do not bear this out.[10] Certainly it is unlikely that the giant pharmaceutical houses would have spent billions of dollars over the years for promotional materials if they did not influence the behavior of doctors. A sign of how much we now rely on mind-altering drugs is the fact that most prescriptions for psychoactive medications are written, not by psychiatrists, but by family doctors and doctors in other specialties.[11] Psychiatry's enthusiasm has influenced physicians to regularly prescribe psychoactive drugs for every emotional ache or pain.[12]

If the "psychopharmacology revolution" has benefited the coffers of the pharmaceutical industry, it has also been a shot in the arm for psychiatry's image. Like other physicians, psychiatrists can now, finally, treat real illnesses with real medicines. As sociologist Andrew Scull has said,

> [Psychiatrists] were given a new treatment modality which enabled them to engage in a more passable imitation of conventional medical practice. In place of acting as glorified administrators of huge custodial warehouses, and instead of relying on crude empirical devices like shock therapy and even cruder surgical techniques like lobotomy to provide themselves with an all too transparent medical figleaf, psychiatrists in public mental hospitals could now engage in the prescription and administration of . . . the classical symbolic accoutrement of the modern medicine man—drugs.[13]

Peter Sterling, a brain researcher at the University of Pennsylvania School of Medicine, has also said,

> In 1954 when chlorpromazine was introduced . . . psychiatry was vulnerable because it suffered from the scorn long heaped upon it by the other medical specialties for having no therapy to offer but "talk" . . . the nation's mental hospitals were bulging . . . "medicine" to treat the insane reinforced the concept that insanity is a medical illness. The drug gave psychiatry a chance to establish decisively its own niche in medicine, and hegemony in the treatment of the insane.[14]

Psychiatry, in other words, has its own reasons for wanting to give so much credit to the new drugs. To the extent that major mental disorders are considered symptoms of brain malfunction, the public is more likely to seek the guidance of psychiatrists, rather than other types of psychotherapists and counselors. This, of course, is what psychiatry stands to gain from the mass marketing of its "biochemical revolution."

The prescribing of a drug requires a medical doctor, and the only medical doctors in the mental health professions are psychiatrists. The more drugs are prescribed, the more psychiatry dominates the field, while other mental health professionals are left to compete for the remainder of the therapeutic dollar.

Out into the Community

Psychiatrists tell us that persons suffering from serious mental disorders, like schizophrenia or major depression, require continued medication after leaving the hospital. The families of these persons often agree: They receive the person back into their midst and are reassured by knowing the person will stay on medication. And some patients agree: They feel more comfortable and secure taking tranquilizers. Many other patients, however, find that the drugs produce more discomfort than relief.

Psychiatry preaches that without these medications, most patients will relapse and require further hospitalization, and countless studies seem to show that this is indeed the case.[15] But these studies have often failed to probe deeply enough. A discharged patient, for example, is strongly pressured to stay on drugs, but often finds their side effects intolerable. He or she refuses to continue the medication and thereby alienates the psychiatrist. The patient may then discontinue contact not only with the psychiatrist but also with the entire mental health system in the community, along with the social support network that backs up the psychiatrist's recommendations. And it is this social support network that is all-important to the patient's regaining and maintaining the ability to live in the community; indeed many of these persons cannot cope without social and emotional support.

Psychiatry prefers not to focus on these factors; rather it insists relapses are caused primarily by cessation of drugs. Once the decompensated person is back in the hospital, and begins to improve, the psychiatrist credits this improvement entirely to the renewal of medication. Overlooked is the fact that in many cases simply being housed for a few days or weeks in a sheltered environment can lead to improvement.

One of the tragic consequences of this excessive reliance on medication is that persons who might accept psychiatric hospitalization, but who do not want to have psychoactive drugs forced on them, find it difficult to locate a psychiatrist who will honor their decision. Most psychiatrists believe that problems serious enough to justify hospitalization also require drugs, and in amounts determined solely by them. As a result, the disturbed person shuns psychiatry and gets no help at all. This suggests that the policy of forcible drugging, by driving away many who want and need help, may actually be contributing to more mental disorder than it prevents.[16]

Side Effects

Why are the major tranquilizers disliked by so many mental patients? What do they actually do to the body and mind? Let's listen to Wade Hudson, a former mental patient turned mental health reform activist, describe his drug experience to a United States Senate committee:

After ten days or so, the effects of the Prolixin*

---

*Prolixin is the brand (trade) name for fluphenazine, a drug closely related to chlorpromazine. Both belong to the same class of tranquilizer—the phenothiazines—that is commonly used in the treatment of psychosis (schizophrenia).

began building up in my system and my body started going through pure hell. It is very hard to describe the effects of this drug and others like it. That is why we use strange words like zombie. But in my case, the experience became sheer torture.

Different muscles began twitching uncontrollably. My mouth was like very dry cotton no matter how much water I drank. My tongue became all swollen up. My entire body felt like it was being twisted up in contortions inside by some unseen wringer. And my mind became clouded up and slowed down.

Before, I had been reasoning incorrectly but at least I could reason. But most disturbing of all was that I feared that all of these excruciating experiences were in my mind, or caused by my mind, a sign of my supposed wickedness.[17]

Another patient described a different set of reactions:

I had a complete inability to concentrate, to read, to write or to think. You become confused, dissipated into the atmosphere around you . . . There is a total disintegration of the self. You have no emotions. You do not feel human. If someone were run over by a car, I probably would not have even reacted to it.[18]

Not only the mind, but also the body is greatly altered by "antipsychotic" drugs.[19] These side effects are routinely dismissed as trivial by psychiatrists, but can be highly upsetting to patients. For instance, vision becomes blurred, so reading is difficult or impossible. Muscles quiver and sometimes ache and go into spasm. A day in the sun may prove quite painful, since the skin becomes hypersensitive. Profoundly disturbing is a common symptom known as akathisia, in which the person experiences a constant restlessness.[20] He or she cannot sit still, and much of the incessant pacing seen on psychiatric wards is the result of this drug-induced condition. Outside the ward, this kind of behavior is often considered by others to be a sign of mental disorder instead of a drug side effect. In men, the breasts may swell (gynecomastia) and ejaculation may be difficult or impossible. In women, the breasts may produce a milky fluid (galactorrhea) and menstrual periods may become irregular.

Sudden death from phenothiazines is a bigger problem than psychiatry dares to admit.[21] Several factors come together to render this possible in a previously healthy patient. First, these drugs are known to increase the likelihood of epileptic seizures; in a seizure a head injury from a fall is a possibility. Next, these drugs lower blood pressure (postural hypotension) and thereby make fainting spells more likely. Again, a head injury is a real possibility. But probably the greatest danger comes from the diminished cough reflex brought on by these drugs.[22] In combination with a seizure, a sluggish cough reflex may lead to the inhalation of material vomited from the stomach. This is the conclusion of Frederick Zugibe, medical examiner of Rockland County, New York, who performed autopsies on patients who had died in mental hospitals. He found that death from this cause was fifteen times more likely in mental hospital patients than in general hospital patients.[23]

A complete discussion of possible side effects could easily fill a chapter, but I want to mention just one more in greater detail. During a recent hike in the mountains my companion was a friend of many years and a former medical school classmate. He is now a urologist, and he told me of his experiences as a consultant at a mental hospital. After hearing his story, I asked him to tape record it for me. Here it is.

Concerning urinary retention and phenothiazines, I have had considerable experience over the years as a urologist. Hardly a week goes by that I don't see somebody referred from the mental health unit, usually with a label of chronic schizophrenia, who has been on phenothiazines for years. These people are usually women; they often present not only with urinary retention but also urinary infection which is secondary to the retention problem. Infection is related to the high degree of residual urine these people carry. They don't empty their bladders well, and if you catheterize them after voiding they often have as much in their bladders as they have voided. Their bladders are often of a very large capacity, and it is difficult to treat these people effectively. I don't think I've ever had anybody taken off phenothiazines, although I always suggest that this would be the best course.[24]

Recently a patient of mine, a young man, had become incontinent (inability to hold his urine) because of the long-term use of phenothiazines. After years of hospitalization he was finally released, but when he returned to the community the sight and smell of his urine-soaked pants led those around him to consider him so bizarre that they tried to have him recommitted to a mental hospital.

Another example of "blaming the victim" occurs with the shuffling gait caused by major tranquilizers. The person walks with short, mincing steps and stooped shoulders. The arms are held stiffly at the sides. This appearance only adds to the likelihood that the person will be considered "weird" even if his or her behavior is otherwise quite reasonable.

If despite these side effects the medication truly exerted an "anti-psychotic" effect, one would think that more patients would welcome these drugs. A psychotic episode is certainly something patients very much want to avoid, not only because it is accompanied by a great deal of emotional pain but also because of the hostile reaction of those around them. Yet a major problem faced by psychiatrists is the "resistant" patient who stops taking the medication at the first opportunity. With few exceptions, psychiatrists say resistance is part of the patient's mental illness. Schizophrenics are too sick to know they need help, and their failure to continue medication is due to "paranoid" thinking or some other type of disordered reasoning.

This argument was accepted for a long time, since the opinions of mental patients were rarely taken seriously. Gradually, however, psychiatrists have been forced to admit that patients resist powerful drugs because they create side effects that even "schizophrenics" cannot ignore.[25] Tragically this begrudging recognition did not come until thousands of patients had been permanently injured. Even worse, patients continue to be subjected to the possibility of permanent drug-induced brain injury even though psychiatrists are well aware that a significant percentage of patients will be harmed in this way. I am talking about a condition called tardive dyskinesia.

The Permanent Brain Injury of Tardive Dyskinesia

For three decades, ever since the phenothiazines were introduced in 1954, countless numbers of mental patients have been the victims of tardive dyskinesia.[26] As a result of permanent damage to portions of the brain known as the basal ganglia and substantia nigra, the patient shows rhythmic smacking and licking of the lips, sucking and chewing movements of the mouth, protrusion of the tongue, and grimacing. In some cases the bizarre movements involve the extremities as well.

Several features of this drug-induced disorder are tragic.

First, the involuntary movements are so bizarre that many people consider them signs of mental illness, rather than a drug side effect. This, in fact, is why psychiatrists ignored the condition for so long. Just as with the restless fidgeting, pacing, and shuffling gait brought on by these drugs, the odd facial movements of tardive dyskinesia were not recognized as drug induced. They were considered part of the patient's schizophrenia.

Second, the involuntary movements may not occur until the drug dosages are lowered or the drug is stopped altogether. As long as the drug is maintained, the brain damage proceeds but the signs are masked. This, of course, makes for greater brain damage before the process is recognized.

Perhaps most troubling of all is that when some patients are either taken off major tranquilizers or given reduced dosages, the now unmasked tardive dyskinesia may be incorrectly diagnosed as a worsening of their schizophrenia. The result? Psychiatrists will view the patient's "relapse" as an indication for *more* medication and additional evidence that patients inevitably relapse without medication.

As George Gardos and Jonathan Cole have commented, "Some patients who appear to deteriorate within a few weeks of drug withdrawal may in fact be developing dyskinesia."[27] In their own study, Gardos and Cole found that "four of the first five" patients diagnosed as experiencing a "relapse" of their schizophrenia were experiencing "increased dyskinetic movements" as a result of drug withdrawal. Putting the patients back on a major tranquilizer amounts, then, to another round of brain injury in the name of treating mental disorder.

Psychiatry has, of course, finally been forced to admit that psychoactive drugs can indeed be dangerous. Psychiatrists still insist, however, that for major mental disorders, drugs are a must. Serious diseases call for serious remedies, psychiatrists argue, and major side effects are the price the patient must pay. Psychiatry prefers to search for yet other drugs to counteract tardive dyskinesia rather than seriously question the need for patients to stay on these drugs indefinitely. Psychiatry is also quite willing, with help from an innovative pharmaceutical industry, to do whatever is necessary to get patients to take their drugs, as a full-page drug advertisement in a psychiatry journal proclaims:

> WARNING: Mental patients are notorious DRUG EVADERS.
>
> Many mental patients cheek or hide their tablets and then dispose of them. Unless this practice is stopped, they deprive themselves of opportunities for improvement or remission, deceive their doctors into thinking that their drugs have failed, and impose a needless drain on their hospital's finances: When drug evaders jeopardize the effectiveness of your treatment program—SPECIFY LIQUID CONCENTRATE.
>
> Liquid concentrate is the practical dosage form for any patient who resists the usual forms of oral medication. It can easily be mixed with other liquids or semisolid foods to assure ingestion of the drug.[28]

New forms of drugs are also colorless, odorless, and tasteless, so patients are not aware that they are being drugged, until they begin to feel the drug's effects on their mind and body. Psychiatrists apparently have no qualms about secretly administering mind-altering drugs, as the drug companies suggest.

At a small private psychiatric hospital, I observed a woman who not only was forcibly hospitalized but also was being drugged without her permission or even her knowledge. According to her records, she suffered from a "paranoid delusion" that someone was poisoning her. The treatment prescribed for this supposed delusion was an increase in the drug she was already receiving. Further on, however, I read that the drug was being given secretly by undetectable placement in her food. It seemed to me quite apparent that she was not delusional at all; rather she was aware that her mind and body were being altered. I could find nothing in the records to indicate that the doctors or nurses had considered this even as a possibility.

These tactics are usually not necessary on a psychiatric ward, because most patients will cooperate even if reluctantly. Those who do resist swallowing pills by trying to cheek them and then later spitting them out are either forced to swallow a liquid preparation or are given the drug by injection. It's a rare patient who will refuse the pills for long, knowing that the alternative is forced injections.

Outside Pressures on Psychiatry to Change

Agencies outside of psychiatry have recently put pressure on psychiatrists to exercise restraint in their use of powerful drugs; these agencies have investigated psychiatry's drug-prescribing habits and found that while the drugs may be new, the reason they are frequently used—for control and management—is not.

For example, the California State Assembly Office of Research found that

> drugs are being prescribed in excessive dosages; some evidence exists that high dosages are for the convenience of the staff. The possibility of neurological impairment, tardive dyskinesia, is greatly increased by high dosages and poor monitoring. Prescribing patterns are frequently irrational.[29]

This study also concluded that

> in both inpatient acute care and care for chronic
> patients, the dangers of the drugs are underesti-
> mated and the effectiveness of the drugs inflated.
> In acute care, medications are often used more
> often than necessary and sometimes too soon after
> admission. Some patients are receiving very high
> dosages early in their treatment, increasing the risk
> of sudden death and other adverse reactions.[30]

The very real dangers of these drugs have been further
documented by California's Department of Health. Responding to public outcry over many unexplained deaths
in the state's mental institutions, the department conducted an investigation of all state mental hospital deaths
between October 1973 and October 1976.[31] The study
found that of all the deaths, "ten percent continued to
pose questions of professional practice or procedural deficiencies." The major cause of these questionable deaths
was excessive medication. Listed as "major problem areas"
were "excessive dosages of psychoactive drugs; failure to
recognize symptoms of overdose; use of medication to
which the patient was allergic; inappropriate choice of
medication; inappropriate polypharmacy;* and failure to
monitor blood drug levels." At Napa State Hospital, the
hospital with more suspicious deaths than any other, it
was found that most of them were caused by "excessive prescribing."

There is every reason to believe that these California
findings are typical of the nation: these data will undoubtedly be duplicated wherever investigations are
undertaken. When Frederick Zugibe reported his findings
showing tranquilizers as a major problem leading to mental
patient deaths in New York, he also "urged . . . that the
review board investigate deaths of patients in all state

---

*Polypharmacy is the practice of giving several drugs at once.

mental institutions because . . . the abuses . . . were endemic to other state facilities as well."[32]

When psychiatry's drug-prescribing habits have been the subject of lawsuits, similar conclusions have been reached. In a number of cases, mental patients have filed suit against the hospitals and doctors holding them, asking the court to call a halt to the indiscriminate use of forced drugging. In each case, the judge decided that while the doctors claimed they used drugs for treatment and treatment alone, the patients were right when they alleged that drugs were being used excessively. In Ohio, U.S. district judge Nicholas Walinski decided in favor of the patients at Lima State Hospital. He noted that the

> widespread use of psychotropic drugs, both in terms of the numbers of patients receiving drugs and the dosages they receive is not, however, necessarily supported by any sound medical course of treatment. Put simply, the testimony at trial established that the prevalent use of psychotropic drugs is countertherapeutic and can be justified only for reasons other than treatment—namely, for the convenience of the staff and for punishment.[33]

In New Jersey, U.S. district judge Stanley Brottman also told the psychiatrists on trial that they were wrong when they claimed that patients were too sick to be allowed the right to refuse medications. He said,

> Only the patient can really know the discomfort associated with side effects of particular drugs . . . it is also difficult for any person, even a doctor, to balance for another the possibility of a cure of his schizophrenia with the risks of permanent disability in the form of tardive dyskinesia.[34]

In Massachusetts, U.S. district judge Joseph Tauro reached similar conclusions. Like Judge Brottman, Tauro told the defendant doctors that while they might know more than the patients knew about drugs, and while the patients might be suffering from serious mental problems, the patients nonetheless had a right to make up their own minds about these drugs. The doctors at Boston State Hospital had argued that "disclosure of the potential side effects of medication may not be in the patient's best interest." Judge Tauro responded:

Although disclosure of the potential side effects of medication may be frightening to the mental patient, this court is not persuaded such a prospect, standing alone, justifies a failure to provide a patient with sufficient information to make an informed treatment decision.[35]

Court decisions have emphasized that the consent of the patient is crucial, regardless of how strongly the doctor believes that the drug will help. This means that *whether the drugs are considered behavior control devices or medical treatment is not the main point.* As the courts have come to recognize in recent years, the fundamental questions regarding forced treatment are ethical rather than medical: Medical acts, very simply, require a patient's consent.

Predicting the Worst

Courtroom decisions have focused primarily on the use of medications on a mental ward, and they leave untouched the largest arena of drug use: the community. The belief that many patients must stay on medication for life represents perhaps the most profound change in psychiatric practice during the past two decades, and is linked to a distorted concept of prevention. Most psychiatrists have come to believe that like doctors who control diabetes with insulin or heart failure with digitalis, they too can prevent recurrence of mental disorders with psychoactive drugs.

One former patient who was told to stay on drugs for life relates what happened to him after he was diagnosed a manic-depressive.

> I was told upon . . . discharge that if I did not take 1500 mg. of lithium per day I would freak out again . . . Because I believed that I had contracted a "mental illness" caused by a "biochemical imbalance," I was strongly inclined not to question my treatment in the hospital or to disagree with the diagnosis laid on me.[36]

This is exceedingly common, and in many cases the psychiatrist's dire warnings are enough to ensure compliance. Still, many patients dislike the drugs so much that they refuse to take them. To counteract resistance, long-acting preparations have been developed. For patients labeled schizophrenic "depot tranquilizers" are used. Suspended in an oily substance that the body absorbs slowly, the depot drug need only be injected every week or two. Once inside the person's body, it continues to work regardless of the person's wishes.

Many psychiatrists consider long-acting drugs to be the wave of the future. As Frank Ayd, a leading authority, has written:

> More and more psychiatric patients will be treated with long-acting oral and injectable preparations . . . Of necessity, mental health care professionals will resort to pharmacotherapeutic regimens that enable them to care for the largest number of patients in the most convenient, expeditious, and economical way feasible. There is every reason to predict that pharmacotherapy with long-acting oral and injectable drugs will escalate.[37]

Heinz E. Lehmann, who helped introduce chlorpromazine to the United States, praises depot drugs by comparing them with contraceptives.

The "pill" works fine as long as it is taken regularly, but as everyone knows, particularly people working in undeveloped countries, it is sometimes very difficult to get the cooperation of the women to really take their pill . . . the intrauterine devices offer much better protection for these women. In a way, we might compare the long-acting chemical preparations of anti-psychotic drugs to the intrauterine devices. Once the medicine is in, the patient is safe for a certain period of time.[38]

In the same article, published in 1970, Lehmann even suggested police intervention to ensure compliance. Lamenting that "we have no legislation that forces anyone to undergo drug therapy outside a mental hospital," he urged laws authorizing police to seek out and apprehend a patient who fails to show up every week or two for injections and to bring the person to a hospital, if necessary by force.

Clinics now exist for the main purpose of giving long-acting tranquilizer injections. Jonas Robitscher, one of the few psychiatrists to speak out against this activity, has called this the "ultimate in impersonal and controlling treatment that can be given to large numbers of patients without any emphasis on the patient as an individual."[39]

But what about the many ex-patients who never show up at a clinic, and stop taking their drugs altogether? For many, the law intervenes.

Court-Ordered Drugging

Long-term medication may be forced on a person through a conservatorship. At a conservatorship hearing, a judge decides (in theory at least) if the person, by reason of mental disorder, is unable to care for himself or herself. Most conservatorship hearings are cursory affairs, in which the judge usually accepts the advice of psychiatrists and local officials. A conservator is appointed, most often a county official with many persons to supervise. The conservator is usually told by psychiatrists to make sure the person stays on the medication. If the person refuses, the conservator has the legal power to force him or her to report to a clinic for a long-acting injection or face rehospitalization.

In many cases the conservator does not need to invoke legal threats to keep the person on drugs. Many patients by this time accept them without any fuss. For those who resist, the doctor's aura of authority is often enough to guarantee compliance. Many patients believe continued medication is virtually required if they are to receive their monthly disability check. Millions of these persons are in a marginal economic position, so they have no wish to antagonize psychiatrists and caseworkers. The patient may be free of a mental hospital, but he or she is still tightly controlled by drugs as well as county officials.

Misinformation

While great numbers of mental patients are forced to stay on drugs, many others do so because they have been told the drugs are necessary for their body chemistry. Many people taking lithium, for example, have told me that this substance is a normal part of the body and that they are manic-depressive because they have a lithium deficiency. Their doctor, they said, had discovered the deficiency through a blood test and had prescribed a lifetime of lithium to correct this abnormality. This idea was expressed to me most recently while I was on a radio talk show. After I mentioned that in psychiatry there are no clear-cut tests to decide which diagnosis best fits a patient, a caller said, "Manic-depressives can be diagnosed by a forty-dollar blood test. Doctors can tell by the lithium level in the blood if the person is manic-depressive or not. It's an absolute, positive test. The doctor can then put in lithium and bring it back to normal level." I explained to the caller that lithium does not occur naturally in the body, so no person has ever suffered "lithium deficiency." The blood test, I continued, was to check the lithium level *after* it had been prescribed by a doctor.

So many patients have told me similar stories that I now know that psychiatrists and family doctors are disseminating a great deal of misinformation about lithium. Authorities advocate that patients be "educated in the concept that lithium is a perpetual preventive much like insulin."[40] These authorities also repeatedly call lithium a "simple, naturally occurring" substance. It therefore comes as no surprise that many patients consider lithium to be like a new vitamin. Unfortunately they are wrong: Lithium is a very toxic substance whose side effects include permanent kidney and thyroid damage, as well as other potential complications.[41]

Similar distortions are being foisted on patients taking "antipsychotic" and "antidepressant" drugs. First, the patient is led to believe that research has shown that major mental disorders are biochemical in origin. Next, the patient is given the equally misleading information that studies show that the drug corrects the abnormality. While many psychiatrists believe these claims will eventually be validated, as of now they remain wishful thinking.[42]

These claims sometimes reach ludicrous proportions. A patient called Sandra, for example, was admitted to the Metabolic Depression Unit of the New York State Psychiatric Institute and put on lithium. Later the sodium level in her blood was measured and found to be elevated. Psychiatrist Ronald Fieve, a leading lithium advocate, writes in his book *Moodswing: The Third Revolution in Psychiatry*, that "in Sandra's case lithium caused a shift in sodium from inside the red cells to the blood plasma and urine. Thus, we concluded that an electrolyte defect of *too much sodium within the cells* [emphasis added] may have been causally related to her depression."[43]

This is truly absurd reasoning. Fieve makes the *assumption* that prior to the dosage of lithium, the sodium in the red blood cells was too high. He does this so that when the sodium comes pouring out of the cells once lithium is given, this can be seen as a "treatment." In fact he has no reason whatsoever to assume the sodium level was too high. On the contrary, the lithium has *injured* Sandra's red blood cells, resulting in the leakage of the normal sodium from the cells. Fieve, like so many of his colleagues past and present, has with the stroke of the pen converted a toxic effect into a medical treatment. As a result, Sandra is the victim of what I believe to be a major abuse. She has been told that she has a defect that in fact does not exist. If she agrees to stay on lithium, her consent will be based on false information. In Sandra's case, consent obviously does not represent a free decision based on accurate information.

The current enthusiasm for lithium illustrates in another way just how determined psychiatry is to promote a medical image, even at the risk of putting the cart before the horse. When it comes to "manic-depressive illness," psychiatry has gone so far as to develop a treatment first and then increase the rate of diagnosis of cases to which the treatment, supposedly an exciting breakthrough, can be applied. When lithium was first made available to physicians in the United States in 1970, manic-depression was rarely diagnosed. Once lithium became popular, more and more patients were "discovered" to have this condition. What was only a few years ago a rare disorder is now widespread.

What's happening? Psychiatry answers that its diagnostic skills are now improved. Manic-depressives were formerly misdiagnosed as schizophrenics, psychiatry says. Nonetheless, even a leading psychiatrist in the drug revolution has admitted that before psychiatrists could diagnose manic-depression in significant numbers, "it required

the introduction of an effective prophylactic treatment."
"We can accept it now," he continued, "because finally
we can do something about it."[44]

Psychiatrist V. Siomoupoulis has also commented on
this epidemic of manic-depression. He writes:

> the recent increase in the number of patients diag-
> nosed as suffering from manic-depressive illness . . .
> perhaps the advent of lithium treatment, and psy-
> chiatry's current emphasis on biological causes and
> treatments, have produced a tendency to overdiag-
> nose manic-depressive illness.[45]

Siomoupoulis reviewed the records of thirty patients diagnosed as manic-depressive. He found:

> Many patients had been diagnosed as manic-depres-
> sive and treated with lithium despite little evidence
> to justify either the diagnosis or treatment. There
> were similar findings among patients referred to us
> by other psychiatric centers.[46]

Finally, Siomoupoulis lamented that "these patients may
continue receiving this highly toxic drug for a long time."

Writing on a different subject, agoraphobia, psychiatrist Robert Seidenberg and attorney Karen DeCrow have
commented on how a popular psychiatric treatment may
"require" a diagnosis fitting that treatment.

> The remedy prescribes diagnosis. When we shape
> diagnosis according to the weapons that are easiest
> to use, "diagnosis proceeds from the available rem-
> edy." Allowing the availability of remedy to dictate
> diagnosis "results in the gross oversimplification of
> deeply rooted problems." Who can doubt that
> psychiatry today suffers from the same malady?[47]

It is strange medicine, indeed, when the incidence of
what is said to be a medical illness depends upon the avail-

ability of a treatment. This practice is the result of psychiatry's eagerness to become a respected medical specialty. Disturbed feelings and disturbing behavior become "diseases" for which new drug treatments are the answer.

Drugs certainly influence the brain, and may therefore influence behavior, but this proves nothing about the nature of mental disorders. Even leading advocates of psychiatry's drug revolution sometimes admit that mental disorders have not been shown to result from faulty brain chemistry. Solomon Snyder, for example, concludes his book *Madness and the Brain* with a frank admission. After reviewing the drugs used both experimentally and for the treatment of schizophrenia, he comments, "No specific biochemical abnormality has ever been demonstrated in the body fluid or brains of schizophrenics."[48]

Can it be said that even if mental problems are not brain diseases, drugs may still help? Quite possibly. But in my view drugs can benefit a person only if the root causes of emotional breakdown are confronted. Help may involve many things, from counseling to social and economic support and possibly to drugs. But at whatever level the problems are approached, reliance on medications hardly seems the answer. Yet today psychiatrists all too often put their primary emphasis on arriving at the "right combination" of mind-altering drugs.

This is nothing new for psychiatry. Over and over psychiatry has developed new ways to alter the bodies of mental patients, and therefore change behavior and feelings, claiming that these alterations proved that a medical disease was being treated. Two hundred years ago, bleeding worked because madness resulted from too much blood in the brain. Only forty years ago lobotomy worked because it corrected disordered circuits in the frontal lobes of the brain. Now drugs supposedly treat as yet undefined brain diseases that cause mental breakdown.

Let us step back from the controversy over whether mental disorders are true medical diseases. In one crucial respect it makes no difference who is right, for in either case the patient should be the one to decide whether to use a medication recommended by a psychiatrist. Yet today, we continue too often to deny this right to mental patients. Let us consider, therefore, the laws and customs that grant the psychiatrist, not the patient, the power to control what may be done in the name of treatment.

CHAPTER 8

INVOLUNTARY PSYCHIATRY AND THE RULE OF LAW

Involuntary hospitalization and treatment of a mental patient is called civil commitment. Psychiatrists are given the legal authority to impose treatment, subject to state laws. This chapter deals with how this authority is regulated. What are the rules? Are they fair? Are they based on realistic appraisals of psychiatry? Or are they based on misconceptions about mental patients and about what psychiatry can and cannot do? Finally, are these rules followed, or are they frequently ignored?

Help for the Patient

The laws that authorize a psychiatrist to make a civil commitment go back centuries—in our country to the very beginning of the Republic, in Europe to the seventeenth century.[1] These laws have always reflected society's attitude toward mentally disordered persons. Civil commitment has traditionally been justified as a benevolent intervention intended to help those unable to help themselves. In legal terms, treatment is part of the state's *parens patriae* (state as parent) powers.[2] Because civil commitment was seen in this benevolent light, for a long time mental hospitals were virtually unregulated by outside agencies. The assumption was that the professionals working at the institution would help and protect the patients. Doctor knew best.

Today everyone agrees that these assumptions were not justified. Patients were often not protected, but rather victimized.[3] They were subjected to a fantastic variety of physical abuses, each one labelled a treatment despite its frequently punishing nature. Dunking, spinning, cooling, heating, toxic chemicals, lobotomy, various shock treatments—the list goes on and on.[4] Patients were absolutely powerless to resist. Entrance to the asylum was often a one-way street. Apathy and hopelessness soon rendered the person even less capable of independent functioning than before.

As a medical student, I first saw how loosely worded civil commitment laws could be used to sweep the streets clean of bothersome persons. As part of a beginning course in psychiatry, I and several others were taken to Chicago's Cook County Courthouse in 1963. In a room next to the jail two doctors spent the morning interviewing the skid row alcoholics who had been arrested the night before. Only one doctor was a psychiatrist, and he clearly dominated the procedure. Each interview lasted only a few minutes, yet in those few minutes a man was either released or committed to the state asylum. In each case, the psychiatrist asked a few routine questions, mostly concerning where the person lived and how he took care of himself. Sometimes the doctor seemed to lead the person with questions like, "What have the voices been telling you?" Whenever a person was unable to answer in a way that satisfied the doctor, he was certified as "mentally ill and in need of treatment." These words fulfilled the legal requirements for indefinite confinement in a state asylum. Even to naive medical students, it was a glaring example of naked and unchecked power.

This practice, repeated hundreds of times each day across the country, eventually made it clear that no matter how much we might talk about "helping" the mentally disordered by confining them in institutions, the procedure was badly in need of reform. Too many people were being locked up for too long with virtually no attention paid to their civil rights. Critics began to talk openly about asylums that have always existed as much for the convenience of the community as for the good of the individual. By the 1960s, even those in charge—the psychiatrists— were ready to admit that a change was necessary.[5] Summing up this widespread recognition, Alan Stone, Harvard professor of law and psychiatry and president of the American Psychiatric Association in 1979–80, wrote that society was simply using mental hospitals to confine "unwanted people cheaply."[6]

Protection for Society

Slowly, a few states began to pass new civil commitment laws, beginning with California in 1967. These new laws focused more attention on the person's right to be left alone, instead of focusing exclusively on the doctor's opinion that "treatment" was needed. Out of this trend came an emphasis on "dangerousness." The laws now proclaimed that persons considered a danger to themselves or to others could be civilly committed to a mental hospital; persons mentally disordered but not dangerous to themselves or to others could not be confined. The new laws also promised greater protection for those already confined in a mental institution. In place of indefinite confinement, which sometimes amounted to a life sentence, a periodic review was required. Release was to follow as soon as a person was no longer considered a danger.

This shift from "indefinite" commitment laws to "danger period" laws is still taking place. Most states have now adopted the new criteria, and in 1975 the U.S. Supreme Court added its voice. Kenneth Donaldson had been confined in a Florida asylum for fifteen years, despite the fact that he had never hurt himself or anyone else. The high court finally ordered him released, writing that

a finding of mental illness alone cannot justify a state's locking a person up against his will and keeping him indefinitely in simple custodial confinement . . . There is no Constitutional basis for confining such persons involuntarily if they are dangerous to no one and can live safely in freedom.[7]

The Court's ruling sounded highly progressive, and was indeed a step in the right direction. But no sooner did this idea gain ground than some apparently unrelated events once again raise profound questions about a psychiatrist's power to lock up a mental patient. For who, after all, is in a position to know which persons are dangerous and which are not? Most people assumed that if anyone could know, the psychiatrist could. When a New York prisoner named Johnnie Baxstrom tried to get out of prison, the assumption that "psychiatrists can predict dangerousness" was finally proved false.

Operation Baxstrom

While Baxstrom was serving his two-year prison sentence for assault, he was transferred to Dannemora State Hospital, one of New York's asylums for the criminally insane. He was considered by psychiatrists to be dangerously mentally ill; when his sentence expired, he was not released. His status was simply switched from prisoner to patient. He now faced indefinite confinement under the civil commitment laws, and this might last a lifetime.

At that time, 1961, there was nothing illegal about this action; the same thing had been done to many other prisoners. Challenging the state's right to make him into a mental patient without any legal hearing, Baxstrom eventually came before the U.S. Supreme Court.[8] The Court decided in 1966 that once a prisoner had completed his term, he could not be further confined by administrative fiat. Before a person could be civilly committed, a hearing must take place, at which the person might be able to prove that commitment was not justified.

As a result of this ruling, nearly one thousand persons confined in maximum security prison-hospitals were transferred to ordinary mental hospitals. This mass transfer became known as Operation Baxstrom. In an attempt to determine the accuracy of psychiatric predictions of dangerousness, researchers could for the first time follow the progress of a person—outside of prison—whom psychiatrists had considered too dangerous for such a transfer. Until Operation Baxstrom, any prisoner considered dangerous was kept in strict confinement, leaving no opportunity for the inmate to demonstrate if he or she would be dangerous in the freer setting of a mental hospital or even in the community. Would those labeled dangerous but nonetheless given greater freedom by the Supreme Court's decision, the researchers could now ask, in fact turn out to be a threat?

When the results were evaluated, they were devastating, primarily because so many research teams came up with the same conclusions. Psychiatrists were totally unable to correctly identify the dangerous and the nondangerous.[9] The results should have sent shock waves through the legal and psychiatric communities. Prisoners were not the only ones being confined because a psychiatrist had labeled them dangerous. Each year, under the new civil commitment laws, thousands of patients were being forced to remain on mental wards for the same reason—danger to self or others.[10]

Perhaps because Operation Baxstrom exposed a major weakness at the very core of psychiatry's special status— the authority to treat patients through the civil commitment process—psychiatry ignored these findings. It was only later that psychiatry emphasized its problem with predicting dangerousness, when psychiatry was required to protect itself financially and professionally.

The Murder of Tatianna Tarasoff

In 1969, Prosenjit Poddar, a student at the Berkeley campus of the University of California, told his psychotherapist, Lawrence Moore, that he planned to kill his former girlfriend Tatianna when she returned to school at the end of the summer. She had jilted him and he was determined to get even. The therapist, a psychologist who worked for the university's Student Health Service, tried to get Poddar hospitalized. But when the campus police interviewed Poddar, they did not think he was bizarre in any way and let him go. Later he carried out his threat, stabbing Tarasoff to death.

After learning that Poddar had warned of what he planned to do, Tarasoff's parents sued Poddar's therapist and the university, because no one in their family had been notified of the danger.[11] In response, the American Psychiatric Association (APA) protested that psychiatrists have no examinations to determine whether or not a person is dangerous. If the Tarasoff parents were to win their suit, psychiatrists might be held legally and financially responsible in other cases; a dangerous precedent might be established. Psychiatry now had to show, therefore, that it had no special skills for predicting violent behavior.

To support its contention, the APA presented research literature on psychiatric predictions of dangerousness. In a legal brief submitted to the California Supreme Court, for example, the APA pleaded, "Study after study has shown that this fond hope of the capability accurately to predict violence in advance is simply not fulfilled." Such a prediction was "an impossible burden upon the practice of psychotherapy." "It requires," the APA continued, "the psychotherapist to perform a function . . . he is ill-equipped to undertake; namely the prediction of his patient's potential dangerousness." Finally, the APA flatly denied that "mental health professionals are in some way more qualified than the general public to predict future violent behavior."[12]

After these startling confessions were blurted out in an effort to protect its members' financial future, psychiatry found itself between a rock and a hard place. If psychiatrists were not "more qualified than the general public" to decide who was dangerous, how could society justify the confinement of mental patients on the word of psychiatrists? It would obviously be necessary to find a new way to justify the involuntary hospitalization of mental patients. An alternative had to be found.

If You Don't Thank Us Now, You'll Thank Us Later

Psychiatry's leaders developed an alternative line of reasoning to justify involuntary confinement. From now on, they say, we should ask the psychiatrist to predict, not whether dangerous behavior is likely, but whether after confinement and forced treatment the person will be grateful to us later for having done this. This scheme has been called the Thank You method, even by its inventor, Alan Stone, the Harvard professor and former APA president mentioned above. He has spelled out precisely what the psychiatrist should ponder in deciding whether or not to confine a patient:

> Would a reasonable man, given the patient's serious illness and suffering, be willing to give up a certain amount of freedom in that particular institution in exchange for a treatment that in similar cases produces a specific range of results ... this is the Thank You Theory of Civil Commitment.[13]

This method has not been formally adopted by any state, but it has become an official line advocated by the APA, its district branches, and by local psychiatric societies. In the 1980s, the courts, legislatures, and the general public are being asked to grant psychiatrists the authority to confine a person if there is a "thank you" coming up.

In what cases is delayed gratitude to be expected? According to Stone, those situations in which "illness impair[s] the person's ability to accept treatment."[14] This statement should hardly surprise us. As we have seen, psychiatry has from its beginnings explained the reluctance of mental patients to accept treatment as a symptom of their disorders. Loren Roth, another APA leader, has written, for example, that when a patient refuses hospitalization, he or she may not "understand the generally agreed-upon consequences . . . both of being treated and of not being treated."[15] If we consider psychiatry's track record of past treatments, we might wonder whether refusal indicates that many patients understand all too well the possible consequence of being involuntarily treated.

Based on what I have seen after fifteen years in psychiatry, I have little doubt that the new Thank You scheme, which is in fact a return to a "doctor knows best" attitude, will if enacted into law do nothing to protect mental patients. For regardless of what the civil commitment laws require psychiatrists to certify, they will say or write whatever is necessary to justify the treatment they feel is needed. At a recent symposium, Loren Roth and a lawyer for the APA, Joel Klein, individually told me they knew this to be true. This should not be taken simply as an indictment of psychiatrists. Rather, this behavior is more a response to the enormous pressure placed on them by society than a sign that they enjoy their authority.

The inconsistencies in our civil commitment laws only begin to tell the story. What the rules say and what psychiatrists do are usually two different things.

Ignoring the Law

If the laws governing commitment and treatment were consistently followed, the incidence of abuse of mental patients would be drastically reduced. But the laws are frequently ignored. Indeed all groups of professionals in the mental health system—judges, attorneys, psychiatrists, administrators, social workers, psychiatric nurses and technicians—often ignore the law because they consider the legal limitations merely a formality that need not hinder their work. They see themselves as answering to a higher authority, one that requires the patient to receive treatment no matter what. In private, many psychiatrists are frank in admitting that they care little about what the law says, and will do what they must to treat the patient, regardless of what legislators in the state capital have written into law.

For two years in the early 1970s I was a party to this lawlessness. During that time I was responsible for the crisis intervention unit at a community mental health center in the San Francisco Bay Area. That was before I decided that I would henceforth refuse to participate in any form of involuntary psychiatry. On the crisis unit we often dealt with persons brought to us by force, either by the police or by family members. The crisis unit staff would interview the person and decide whether or not he or she should be held. The individual brought in by police was almost inevitably kept involuntarily, because it was considered bad form to release someone too quickly after the police left. Even though persons were not considered a danger to themselves or others, they were held, often for several days.

The individual brought in by family members was also usually kept involuntarily. This occurred because if we told the family members that we could legally commit persons only found to be a danger to themselves or others,* the tired relatives would become annoyed and exasperated, often demanding commitment. The simpler solution for us

---

*California and most other states permit commitment of those considered "gravely disabled," that is, those unable to provide for their food, clothing, or shelter. This is clearly a form of "danger to self."

was to ignore the provisions of the law and to commit the person anyway. Who would complain? Only the patient, who seldom knew the law; besides, no one gave much credence to patient demands for release.

Our behavior was not exceptional. Indeed, based on my personal experience as a psychiatrist, I would estimate that in no more than one fourth of the cases in which a person is certified as dangerous is there any evidence that that person is really dangerous. It turns out, in other words, that although state legislatures have tightened the laws governing civil commitment, the mental health community is for the most part disregarding them. In most cases, involuntary hospitalization takes place, not because a danger exists, as the law requires, but because the family needs a rest, the psychiatrist believes treatment is necessary, the community feels the person is a nuisance, or some combination of these three. When it comes to protecting mental patients from the state, we have made more progress on paper than in practice.

Research is now coming to light indicating that the mental health system routinely disregards the law. Carol Warren of the University of Southern California reviewed one hundred cases of mental patients asking judges to order their release from the hospital.[16] Hearings were ordered to determine whether the person was unable, because of mental disorder, to provide for food, clothing, or shelter. If so, the law said, the person would be considered "gravely disabled" and kept in the hospital. If not, the person was to be released.

Warren found a pattern of routine disregard for the law. Judges and attorneys were as guilty of this as were the psychiatrists. The patients' lawyers, for example, "refrained from vigorous advocacy of their clients' legal rights." If a patient refused medication, the judge ordered the person to remain in the hospital even though nothing in the law authorized this. Warren concluded that most patients were being held illegally. "Evidence was introduced in one case that an individual's clothing was bizarre, and in another that the petitioner [patient] walked around in various military uniforms." In another example, the person was confined because "her home was dirty." Finally, Warren noted a factor that is seldom recognized by those who write the laws or by the courts that review the laws, but has always been at the heart of why we confine the mentally disordered: The mental hospital was being used as a safety valve for what she called "the relief of family tensions."

If, as Warren's research illustrates, the mental health laws are ignored in court, they are probably heeded even less by the mental hospital admitting psychiatrist. In 1977 the Minnesota Supreme Court commissioned a study of how mental patients get into a hospital in that state.[17] The study found that doctors not infrequently confined patients despite any "direct information about the subject." Incarceration came "upon the request of the persons who bring the subject to the door of the hospital." Here, too, it was a matter of the "relief of family tensions."

The Catch-22 Voluntary Patient

Although I have been speaking of those who are involuntarily committed to a mental hospital, I must emphasize that *of all the persons treated against their wills by psychiatrists, most appear to the outside world to be voluntary patients.* Because few people understand this, most people commonly believe that involuntary psychiatry is much less of a problem now than it used to be. To the contrary, the problem is perhaps bigger than ever, and one reason is that the use of force is more disguised today than it has been in the past. No one could deny, thirty years ago, that state asylum inmates had no say in what treatments they received. But now that most treatment takes place in community clinics or small, private psychiatric hospitals, voluntarism appears on the surface to be the norm. To understand how deceptive this is, we need to consider the emergency room or admissions office of the local psychiatric facility.

The person who resists hospitalization is told that if he or she will not sign "voluntary" admission papers, hospital admission will be accomplished by the use of formal, involuntary commitment papers. The "choice" is left up to the patient, but the doctor makes it clear that he or she will be very displeased if the patient does not sign the papers. According to my observations, in nearly all cases the person will comply. For one thing, the potential patient believes that if he cooperates, he will be dealt with more leniently in the hospital, not realizing that signing a voluntary admission form brings on the worst of both worlds—subjection to whatever the doctor orders, but with fewer protections than are available to the overtly involuntary patient. Why? Because the laws governing psychiatric hospitalization assume that the terms *voluntary* and *involuntary* mean what they say—that is, that an involuntary patient needs protection against possible abuse, whereas a voluntary patient does not need protection because he or she can simply refuse a treatment or leave the hospital. Both of these assumptions, however, are false.

With a voluntary admission form in hand, the psychiatrists feel that they are treading on safer ground, and are therefore freer to do whatever seems best. In his book *How to Survive Being Committed to a Mental Hospital*, former patient Doug Cameron goes to the heart of the matter:

> Based upon my own general experience as an incarcerent, most patients inside a mental hospital are there involuntarily. Technically, or statistically, though, most patients are listed as voluntary. This is because they have signed a voluntary commitment paper. But this is highly misleading since

most of us only sign due to a great amount of pressure from the system.[18]

Cameron also describes the price he paid for his initial unwillingness to become a "voluntary" patient:

> For refusing to take the tranquilizers offered me, and for refusing to sign the "voluntary commitment" papers, I was, instead, whisked away into solitary confinement. Lying there, tied to my bed as I was, many thoughts and feelings passed through my mind. Among the foremost of these feelings were fear and rage, indignation and doubt. Two weeks can be a long time to lay on one's back and stare at a light bulb that never goes out.[19]

Eventually, Cameron agreed to sign the voluntary admission papers.

> This turned out to be the wrong decision, however, because as soon as I signed, I was immediately whisked off and given a long series of shock treatments.[20]

Looking back on the whole affair, Cameron talks about why it is actually safer to be "involuntary" rather than "voluntary."

> Either way, one is not going to get out until the doctor says, but the great advantage of being there *involuntarily* is that if the doctor does decide to use shock or whatever, then you know and the doctor knows that you have a greater chance against him in a court of law afterwards in case you feel there has been malpractice. Contrarily, if one signs a voluntary commitment paper, hoping to be rewarded for one's cooperative behavior, then one's chances of getting shock or whatever are actually greater than if one hadn't cooperated . . . the doctor can always point out that one "volunteered"

for "treatment" . . . even though in reality the doctor may have given you the treatment against your will.[21]

During the years I worked at a community mental health facility, I observed that for every formally involuntary admission there were several formally voluntary admissions that were coerced signings, whereby the persons were forced to remain in the hospital and be treated against their will. *Lack of understanding of this process is one of the major obstacles to meaningful reform of the mental health system.*

Two "Voluntary" Patients

Let us consider the example of a young woman I shall call Nan.[22] I met her while preparing to testify before a legislative committee in support of a bill to tighten the consent procedures for electroshock treatment. Nan told me she had received electroshock against her will. When her private psychiatrist told her to enter a psychiatric hospital for shock treatment, she reluctantly agreed. After entering the hospital, however, she changed her mind. Despite her protests, she was given shock treatment and experienced the usual effects of confusion and memory loss. After a few shocks, however, her wish to stop the treatment became so strong that she said to a nurse, "I just have to get out of here. I'm leaving no matter what you say." It was then that she escaped.

When the psychiatrist who had sent her to the hospital found out that Nan had run away, he telephoned her at home and said he would call the police if she did not return to the hospital. Under this pressure she returned, telling the nurses, "I really don't want to be here; I feel like I'm being forced to have shock. The doctor said if I didn't come back he'd send the police after me." Despite these events, her readmission was called voluntary, with no mention of her documented fear of shock treatment, of her desire not to be in the hospital, or of the threat of police intervention. She received more shock treatment during her second hospitalization, until she fled once more.

This kind of behind-the-scenes involuntarism is as typical of today's psychiatry as were yesterday's strait-jackets. Consider the experience of another "voluntary" patient. A thirty-five-year-old man, whom I will call Bill, was admitted to a psychiatric hospital after a phone conversation between his estranged wife and the psychiatrist who arranged the admission. Bill had been drinking and ingested a small number of Valium tablets, apparently hoping that this suicide gesture would bring his wife back to him. She instead asked the local psychiatrist to have Bill admitted to a psychiatric hospital. He agreed to go, but once on the ward found that the doors were locked behind him. Immediately he decided to leave, but when he tried to he was forcibly given an injection of a major tranquilizer. In his hospital records I noted that this attempt at escape was charted as "restlessness."

When the effects of the drugs wore off, Bill renewed his attempts to leave. For his efforts he was rewarded with another injection and strapped in bed with leather restraints. He struggled to release himself, and by 2:30 A.M. had "apparently chewed right wrist restraint." When this was discovered, the restraints were reapplied and he received yet another forced injection.

Bill had not yet met with a psychiatrist, but already shock treatment was scheduled to begin the next morning. By the time two treatments had been given, he was, according to nurses' notes, unable to hold his urine, having bowel movements in bed or on the floor, and totally unable to eat without assistance. He was, in other words, reduced to an infantile state by the brain injury of the shock treatment. The psychiatrists called his confusion and memory impairment "therapeutic." They said he was "doing well at present" and was "less restless." The nurses also noted that he "takes medication without any persuasion but he asks what it is for." He was "pleasant on approach." The shock treatment was obviously having the desired effect.

The next day, Bill received no shock and his brain began to recover enough for him to understand what was happening. He again tried to escape, and again was given forced injections for "increasing agitation and elopement precaution." Shock was resumed the next morning, but even this did not stop him now. According to his hospital records,

> when door being opened to let other patients in, patient pushed way through the door and ran down the steps. Orderlies called to exits. Followed patient to parking lot. Forcibly carried patient to hospital, placed on stretcher, and returned to room. Placed in five-point restraint.

Another injection controlled him that night, but by morning he "seemed to be getting restless, begging to get out of restraints. Sodium amytal given for increased restlessness." Later that morning, still in leather restraints, he was again given shock. That afternoon the following was noted in his hospital record: "Had electric razor—told his wife he was going to cut his restraints but gave it to her with no difficulty." The shock treatment so confused Bill that he mixed up an electric razor with a razor blade. When nurses tried to place him in restraints that night, a fight ensued. He bit a security guard who was trying to subdue him. He was then kept in restraints continuously for the next three days.

During this entire nightmare, Bill was classified as a voluntary patient. Upon admission, he had signed a voluntary admission form, and the forced injections, shock treatment, and leather restraints were part of his "voluntary" treatment.

Eventually Bill managed to telephone a lawyer, who began to put some pressure on the hospital.* The psychiatrist's immediate response was to ask one of his colleagues to examine Bill and see if he was suitable for "involuntary" commitment. With formal commitment papers in place, Bill and his lawyer would have to go to court to get a release. This new doctor noted Bill's confusion and disorientation, but chose to ignore the obvious fact that the electroshock treatment had caused it. Instead, he diagnosed the signs of the shock-induced brain syndrome as signs of mental illness and concluded that Bill was indeed an appropriate prospect for involuntary commitment.

A few days later, the psychiatrist and the hospital decided to release Bill rather than go through a court fight. Before his release, he received one more shock treatment. Upon discharge, he was described as "forgetful and confused but cooperative." My review of his records made it clear that only the presence of the lawyer kept him from being held even longer and receiving even more shock as a "voluntary" patient.

Without the hospital records, which were only obtained through his attorney's insistence, no one would be able to understand what had really occurred. The courts and the outside world in general might well brush off Bill's version of the story as the exaggerations of a former mental patient. And because memory is so impaired by shock treatment, he might *not even remember how and why all this had happened to him.* He might see his signature on the hospital admission form, but still wonder why he consented to the very things he had always feared.

Most patients in mental hospitals do not spend their days in leather restraints as Bill did, and most do not receive shock treatment, but his story nonetheless illustrates

_____
*It was this lawyer who sent me Bill's records months later when a lawsuit was pending.

how few protections a supposedly voluntary patient may actually have. To be a voluntary patient would seem to imply that the person has the freedom to leave, for that is certainly the case with hospitalized medical and surgical patients. But a patient who enters a psychiatric ward often discovers that leaving is not as easy. *Despite a patient's status as "voluntary," discharge is contingent upon a doctor's permission.*

Consider the example of Hawaii, whose civil commitment law of 1976 is considered in mental health circles to be progressive.[23] A voluntary patient, the law states, may leave a psychiatric hospital, but only if the doctor decides that the patient is "sufficiently improved so that hospitalization is no longer desirable." Should the doctor feel that "discharge would be dangerous to the patient or to others, proceedings for involuntary hospitalization must be initiated as soon as possible." The voluntary patient may not be allowed to leave, because the psychiatrist may at any time place the person on involuntary status. In classic Catch-22 fashion, a person is voluntary as long as he or she is willing to stay, but involuntary when he or she wants to leave. I know of no state that handles this issue differently.

The psychiatrist often knows from the beginning that a "voluntary" patient will not be allowed to leave but will say nothing about this, since discussion of this point might be rather awkward. To be honest, the psychiatrist would have to say:

> I'm glad you decided to come into the hospital, Mrs. Jones, because if you hadn't, I would have forced you to. And now that you're a voluntary patient here, I hope you don't decide to leave before I say it's ok, because if you do, then I'll have to keep you on as an involuntary patient.

Lifetime Control

After they are released from the hospital, patients may still be coerced into receiving "voluntary" treatment. For while they are often told by their psychiatrists to keep taking their medications indefinitely, many patients stop taking them at the first opportunity. This, as we saw in the last chapter, is because of unpleasant and sometimes disabling effects and side effects. But if a person does this, a conservator may be appointed, and the conservator has the legal authority to ensure that the person complies with whatever treatment the psychiatrist recommends.

The most disturbing aspect of the conservatorship process is its lawlessness. The requirements of the law are simply ignored by all concerned. Specifically, state laws require that the proposed conservatee be unable, because of mental disorder, to provide for basic survival needs, like food, clothing, and shelter. Because psychiatrists usually believe so strongly that psychiatric drugs are essential to the patient's well-being, in many cases doctors equate refusal to take the drugs with a need for conservatorship. There is nothing in the law to permit this, but judges usually go along with little fuss.

Unlike the earlier practice of indefinite commitment to an asylum, a conservatorship must be renewed by a court on a regular basis. State laws even require the state to prove the need for continued control. But once again, the gap between theory and practice is enormous. Take, for example, the systematic abuse found by the Alameda County, California, Legal Aid Society when it investigated how conservatorships were being renewed. Instead of a hearing being held, in which the person's current abilities were judged, a printed form signed by two doctors was routinely submitted to the court. The courts simply rubber-stamped the form and the conservatorship was renewed for another year.

Even when patients did their best to force the system to grant them a real hearing, it did not always take place. According to the Legal Aid Society investigation, "Sue Roe"

> was detained at Napa State Hospital and communicated in writing and through a friend to her public

> defender her wish to vigorously contest any re-
> commitment. Nevertheless, the public defender
> did not contact the individual regarding her pres-
> ence at the recommitment hearing, did not file a
> request for a hearing, and submitted her case . . .
> without even informing the individual that her re-
> commitment was to be passed upon or bringing her
> to court.[24]

As this case illustrates, some of those under conservatorship are kept—even today—indefinitely in mental institutions. While this is undoubtedly less common than it was
in the past, commitment to a mental hospital may still last
for many years.

Is what happened to Sue Roe merely an extreme case?
Perhaps. Still, the Legal Aid researchers found that in nine
out of ten cases the conservatorship renewal was not even
filed with the court until after the legal deadline.[25] According to the law, the courts should have rejected every
one of these renewal petitions, freeing each person from
state control. *In not one case was this done.* In one instance, the court renewed a conservatorship over a man incarcerated in a state asylum, even though the doctors were
two and a half months late in their petition for recommit-
ment.[26]

The Legal Aid Society also found that it was not unusual for a person to have a conservatorship renewed, year
after year, on the basis of

> medical summaries which simply repeat the writ-
> ten medical summaries prepared and submitted to
> the court in previous years. In one example, the
> same report was submitted three years in a row,
> except that each year it was signed by a different
> doctor.[27]

University of San Diego law professor Grant Morris has
also studied the conservatorship process, and his findings
are equally startling.[28] Troubled by the fact that in his own

community over half of those persons confined on a "72-hour emergency commitment" were subsequently placed on a conservatorship, Morris began sending his law students to the local San Diego County Superior Court to see what was happening. "The students," Morris writes, "examined the court files in each case."[29] The students immediately noted that conservatorships were being used as a means to force treatment (drugs) on people, whether or not they were in fact "gravely disabled." Morris went on to conclude:

> The definite impression of many data gatherers is that the conservatorship device is used to avoid the necessity of obtaining consent to treatment from recalcitrant patients. One can only speculate on the number of people who are coerced into accepting "voluntary" treatment by a threat to initiate the conservatorship process if the individual is unwilling to accept treatment.[30]

Other highlights of Morris's study include:

— Of forty-five individuals under temporary conservatorship, only four were allowed to remain at home.

— Almost invariably . . . the conservator appointed by the court is an institutional conservator . . . In only one case was a relative—the conservatee's brother—appointed conservator.

— The conservator may place his conservatee in a mental treatment facility only if the court order establishing the conservatorship specifically grants him the authority to do so. In every case studied, the court granted the conservator this placement power—almost invariably, the power is exercised.[31]

Although guardianships and conservatorships are generally thought of as a way to protect the elderly and the infirm, Morris found that nearly 60 percent of the conservatorships were placed on persons under age thirty-six.[32]

If fair hearings led to these outcomes, it might be argued that the conservatorship process was working to protect helpless persons, and not simply as a convenient tool to force long-term drugging. Consequently, Morris's students also studied the nature of the hearings themselves. Some of their findings were:

—The lawyers did not consider themselves advocates in an adversary process.

—Of the sixty-three court hearings observed. . . thirty-six lasted three minutes or less, and only nine hearings lasted nine minutes or longer.

—In forty-two cases (71%) the proposed conservatee's lawyer asked no questions of the reporting psychiatrist. In most of the remaining twenty-one cases, the lawyer asked only one question.

—In only one case did the proposed conservatee's counsel request either the assistance of a psychiatrist or the examination of the proposed conservatee by another psychiatrist. In none of the cases did counsel for the proposed conservatee offer testimony of an independent psychiatrist.

—Only once did a lawyer urge that the proposed conservatee be permitted to retain his drivers license. In no case did the lawyer resist the imposition of contractual disability on his client. Most significantly, in only two cases did the attorney oppose the court's granting the placement power to the conservator.[33]

On the basis of these findings, we can hardly be surprised by Morris's overall conclusion. "In sum," he writes, "the court hearing in the typical conservatorship case is a mere formality, rubber stamping the decisions made earlier by psychiatrists and the conservatorship investigator."[34]

Unfortunately, the problems do not end at this point. What Morris found happening *after* these "trials" was equally disturbing. Once the conservatorship was in place, the person was usually "discharged to nursing homes or board and care homes. A CMH [Community Mental Health] aftercare team circuit-rides to these facilities, interviewing once every two weeks each patient."[35]

A report prepared for the California legislature and the San Diego County Board of Supervisors describes more precisely what "aftercare" really means:

> The primary responsibility of the Aftercare Team is to supervise the patient's medication. The preferred medication is Prolixine [sic], an inject-able which maintains effective blood levels for two weeks or longer. The description of a typical day of activity by the Aftercare Team to a large board and care home consists of interviews with residents for an average of five minutes each by one of the Team's two psychiatrists, a brief entry made in the patient's folder, and the administration of medication by the nurse.[36]

Asked about this, the psychiatrist in charge of the After-care Team confirmed that 80 to 90 percent of the conserva-tees placed in after-care settings received an injection of Prolixin every two weeks. He also admitted to prescribing to some patients six to eight times the maximum dosage recommended by the manufacturers of Prolixin.[37]

Clearly today, just as in the past, mental patients have far fewer rights than the rest of us. And while it is true that many of today's patients are held only a few days in a hospital and then released, it would be a serious mistake to underestimate the effect a short-term stay can have on their lives—often for the worse. A few days of observation and drug treatment may seem mild compared to the classi-cal snake pit horror story, but consider that during this hospitalization a psychiatric dossier is formulated, often filled with exaggerations, distortions, and half-truths. Iron-ically, family members are frequently the source of the one-sided information. The things they say to the hospital psychiatrist may well be influenced by feelings of fatigue and exasperation. Psychiatrists may easily put more faith in the family's information than in what the patient says. Mental patients are not generally given much credibility, especially at the time they are being admitted to a hospital.

Once placed in the hospital record, any information becomes "fact," following the person around for the rest of his or her life. If the ex-patient protests that the "facts" are wrong, his or her opinions are often disregarded by the rest of the world. This stigmatizing may be very damaging. A psychiatric file and a psychiatric diagnosis immediately convey second-class citizenship. Our society, despite rhetoric to the contrary, looks very differently at a psychiatric patient than at a medical patient. Society tends to treat ex-convicts better than ex-mental patients.[38]

For all the talk about "progressive" mental health legislation, some of which has indeed been worthwhile, the core of the problem remains untouched: We as a society continue to believe we need to lock up certain people at certain times, even though they have not broken any law, and we believe that those people will benefit from our doing so. Yet the only help that can truly aid a mentally disordered person is the help that person is willing to accept. Coercive treatment of any sort cannot heal a troubled person.

CHAPTER 9

ABOLISHING INVOLUNTARY TREATMENT

Involuntary psychiatric treatment denies to mental patients basic protection that the rest of us enjoy—protection from unwanted physical interference by the state. Involuntary treatment thus makes mental patients into second-class citizens vulnerable to abuse. In addition, forced treatment denies more help to needy persons than it delivers. For these reasons, I propose that our society abolish the practice of forced commitment and treatment.

This proposal immediately raises many doubts and fears that should be respected and examined. I will try to show that a psychiatry limited to voluntary services would help more people, not fewer. I will also try to show that we need not feel threatened by an end to involuntary treatment.

The Dangerous Mental Patient

Much confusion arises from the failure to distinguish between the terms *dangerous* and *criminal*. *Dangerous* refers to what a person *might* do, whereas *criminal* refers to what a person has already done. Our legal tradition tells us that the state may not presume what a person will do, but must limit its police power to illegal behavior already taken place or imminent. If ordinary citizens may not be incarcerated as "dangerous," why should mental patients be treated differently? If a mentally disordered person commits a crime, he or she should be arrested, as the law instructs for anyone. Mental patients, however, are not

177

particularly prone to criminal behavior.[1] They represent no special threat and we fear them needlessly. We therefore should not allow our prejudices about mental disorder to deny mental patients their full rights of citizenship.

If the mentally disordered are not particularly dangerous, why are we so afraid of them? One answer is sensationalism. In those few violent crimes where the assailant has a history of mental disorder, media stories tend to hastily assume that mental disorder was the "cause." Other reasons, like jealousy, greed, or impulsiveness, make a less interesting story. The result is a recycling of the myth that the mentally disordered are especially prone to violence. The media feed us these stories, and we in turn feed the media by responding favorably and uncritically.

Again, violent behavior is often simply *defined* as crazy. A good example is the frequent comment that "murder is an insane act," or "anyone who commits a murder must be crazy." This establishes the association of mental disorder and violence by fiat. The only evidence of insanity is the crime itself.

Let us consider the person who in October 1982 was lacing Tylenol capsules with cyanide. Since he or she has never been found, no one knows why this was done, or what the killer is like. A good many people, with plenty of help from media stories, nonetheless assumed that the cyanide killer was crazy. In the issue of October 18, 1982, *Time* presented in an essay entitled "The Maniac in the Balance" the inevitable "psychiatric portrait" of the unknown killer. Included were the following insights:

— the murderer is likely to be a loner, isolated and unnoticed, with few if any friends. He is probably low in self-esteem, paranoid and hypersensitive, taking offense at real or imagined slights from those around him.
— unlike the textbook-case mass murderer, who is often a paranoid schizophrenic, the Tylenol killer is appar-

ently not disabled by delusions or incapacitated by
hallucinations.

— the killer is a 'borderline' personality . . . He may undergo
transient psychosis intermixed with healthy intervals.[2]

It is little wonder many believe that mentally disordered
persons are dangerous. But guilty as the media may be,
other factors must be operating, since our fears are older
than the media.

People who suffer a major emotional breakdown (psychosis) may indeed behave irrationally. Few are violent,
but their irrational behavior is nonetheless disturbing and
frightening. Society's traditional response has been to
lock up harmless mental patients. Other persons formerly
considered unpleasant to have around, such as epileptics,
were also institutionalized. They too were considered
dangerous.[3] But once we stopped locking up epileptics,
we realized they were not dangerous. We have yet to recognize that our fears about the mentally disordered are also
groundless.

Not only bizarre behavior, but bizarre speech also
frightens us. Irrational talk may be even more frightening
than ordinary criminal behavior, because the criminal at
least talks straight. When someone speaks irrationally, we
become frightened of possible unpredictability and possible dangerousness. In recent years investigators have
questioned these assumptions linking mental disorder and
dangerousness. Saleem Shah of the Center for Studies of
Crime and Delinquency, a program of the National Institute of Mental Health, has found that studies of the alleged
dangerousness of the mentally ill "do not support the
public stereotype of the mentally ill as highly dangerous
and unpredictable." Shah concluded that "the mentally ill
do not constitute one of the most dangerous groups in our
society."[4]

Our society thus has no rational foundation to believe
public safety will be enhanced by preventively confining

and involuntarily treating the mentally disordered. While fear may be a natural reaction to the irrational behavior of some disturbed persons, society should nonetheless resist the temptation to deprive the mentally disordered of their civil rights. Furthermore, our reliance on coercive psychiatry actually *interferes* with the protection of society. In the case of persons who have been violent and also have a history of mental disorder, it is not unusual for criminal prosecution to be waived in favor of confinement to a mental ward. Instead of being arrested and prosecuted, these persons are conveniently dumped in mental hospitals and heavily drugged. A few days or weeks later, however, they may be on the streets again. Society in this way excuses those few mental patients who commit criminal acts, and punishes (involuntarily treats) the vast majority of mental patients who commit no crimes. This is not a rational way to protect society.

Preventing Suicide

There is no evidence that society reduces suicide through involuntary hospitalization and forced treatment.[5] Sociologist David Greenberg in an extensive review of such efforts has commented, "Less than a handful of controlled studies of the effectiveness of treatment measures have been reported. The results have been either inconsistent or negative."[6] As with allegedly dangerous patients, suicidal patients are being locked up on the undocumented belief that involuntary treatment accomplishes its stated goal.

Psychiatrists are nonetheless expected to use involuntary treatment to prevent suicide. Believing they have little choice but to comply, for fear of lawsuits and criticism of their professional competence, psychiatrists naturally defend these policies. They steadfastly maintain that without involuntary psychiatric treatment suicide rates would increase. Shock treatment is especially touted for suicide prevention.

There is reason to question whether in truth these forced treatments promote rather than prevent suicide. Greenberg has written, "Institutionalization may not prevent suicide, but in fact may result in more suicides than treatment on an outpatient basis . . . Commitment to a mental institution, especially if involuntary, may create additional problems for the patient without alleviating old ones."[7] And psychiatrist Peter Breggin has observed, "Trying forcibly to prevent suicidal activities leads to a struggle between therapist and patient that encourages suicide . . . involuntary treatment and drug therapy humiliate and harm the patient, often causing greater despair and a greater likelihood of suicide."[8]

My own experience as a psychiatrist confirms Breggin's conclusion. I renounced the use of involuntary treatment about ten years ago, even for patients thinking about suicide. I am happy to say that none of my patients has committed suicide. I offer this, not in order to prove that I have greater therapeutic skills than the next psychiatrist, but merely to illustrate that abandoning involuntary treatment hardly means a rash of suicides will result.

There is another way in which our present policies promote suicide. Fear of involuntary treatment keeps depressed persons from psychiatry's doorstep. They stay away. As Breggin comments, "In the absence of involuntary psychiatry, many more of these people might seek help, resulting in an overall greater good."[9] Some of my own patients have reported this attitude. As one recently expressed it, "I could never let them put me back on a psychiatric ward and give me electroshock like they did before. I would kill myself first." I have indeed reviewed the cases of patients who committed suicide rather than face forced admission to a psychiatric hospital.

So far I have been speaking of the truly suicidal patient, but many others are forcibly hospitalized as "suicidal" when their behavior is in fact manipulative: a means to gain attention, a last-ditch effort to keep a partner from leaving, or a way to punish someone. Suicidal manipulations are not to be taken lightly, yet far more harm than good comes from responding with coercive hospitalization. Instead of being helped to confront his or her manipulation, the person is now caught in the "struggle between therapist and patient" described by Breggin. The patient may focus his or her energy on somehow getting out of a locked psychiatric ward instead of working on real problems. Patients may hide from the psychiatrist any feelings that might lead the psychiatrist to delay discharge. Patients frightened of electroshock may put up a good façade, to show the psychiatrist that this treatment is not needed. All these possibilities block the patient from a truly therapeutic relationship with the psychiatrist, for without mutual trust real therapy is impossible.

Pressures on the psychiatrist only magnify these problems. Psychiatrists are expected to use whatever means necessary to prevent suicide, including forced medication, electroshock, and confinement to a "seclusion" room. The doctor, as parent, is responsible for the patient's behavior, and the patient, as child, must be controlled. Psychiatrist Thomas Szasz, a longtime critic of involuntary treatment, has written that

> patients should be deprived of the power to coerce psychiatrists, for example, by the threat of suicide; psychiatrists should be deprived of the authority to coerce patients, for example, by a threat of commitment . . . So long as hospitalized mental patients are regarded as children, and psychiatrists their parents who are largely responsible not only for their welfare but for their conduct toward society as well, the *psychiatrists shall be compelled to exercise autocratic controls over their charges* [emphasis added].[10]

Psychiatrists, moreover, control patients in these situations as much to protect their professional reputations as to save patients' lives. Suicide is a real embarrassment to a psychiatrist—a sign of questionable competence.

I know these feelings from my own experiences practicing psychiatry. Despite my abandonment of forced treatment, I still experience the same emotions as other psychiatrists when faced with the possible suicide of one of
my patients. If the patient ends his or her life, what will
others think of me? Will they believe I could and should
have prevented the suicide? Will the family sue? I frankly
admit that with suicide, I try to talk patients out of it as
much for myself as for them. I doubt that other psychiatrists feel differently. Forced admission to a psychiatric
ward relieves the psychiatrist of these pressures, and so far
few psychiatrists have been willing to forego this easy
path of escape.

Abandonment or Liberation?

Defenders of involuntary psychiatric treatment, particularly psychiatrists, frequently claim a ban on involuntary
treatment would amount to abandoning the mentally ill.
They say far more patients would "die with their rights
on."[11] The experience of being treated against one's will
hardly supports this claim. A ban would be a blessing to
the mentally disordered. As we have seen, mental patients
have all too often been abused by treatments forced on
them. Why has this happened? Because the patients had no
say in their care, not because psychiatrists are malevolent.
Perhaps it is time to ask whether even the most disturbed
mental patients should not be given the choice of avoiding
treatments that so often are damaging.

Many patients have been helped in mental hospitals,
but more have been hurt. Psychiatrist Alan Stone has
written of "the considerable harms that may befall the
individual because of involuntary confinement. These may
include stigmatization, collapse of self-esteem, separation
from family and community, loss of job and impairment of
future employment prospects, as well as, in our current
state of institutional care, a not insubstantial chance of
brutalization or mere physical deterioration in the total

institutions to which many such persons are sent."[12] To these factors we must add the risks of the treatments, particularly drugs and electroshock.

Even for those who seem to benefit, the real question remains: Have they been helped because of involuntary treatment, or in spite of it? Without involuntary treatment, would more or fewer people be helped? By now, it is obvious that my conviction is that abandoning psychiatric force would not mean abandoning mental patients. To the contrary, troubled persons would finally have good reason to trust psychiatry enough to seek help more regularly.

With a totally voluntary system of mental health care, patients could not only trust psychiatrists, they would also find it easier to trust their families. Patients are often afraid of their relatives and may stay away from them for years at a time. This is not merely a sign of their mental disorder but is instead a learned response, for in many cases the family made the decision to have them locked up and treated against their will. Now, they feel that at the first sign of another breakdown, the family may lock them up again. The only way to avoid this possibility is to stay away. If problems recur, the family will not be aware of them and hence will not call the police or the psychiatrist. It is painful to see people avoid the only family they have. With the abolition of forced treatment, this fear, which often remains years after hospitalization, would finally disappear.

Off to Jail?

Most persons treated involuntarily in mental hospitals have done nothing illegal. There is no legal way they could be jailed. The frequent argument that without involuntary treatment masses of mental patients would be jailed is without substance.

Mentally disturbed persons who do commit crimes should be jailed because of their activity, and that alone should determine their length of confinement. If sent to a mental ward instead of a jail, a person guilty of the most minor offense and likely to spend only a few days in jail may instead be placed on a conservatorship.[13] This means control for a year or longer, complete with involuntary use of powerful tranquilizing drugs. Even without a conservatorship, involuntary confinement and drug treatment may easily stretch out for weeks. In essence, the person is punished, not for a crime, but for being mentally disturbed.

The physical conditions in jail are undoubtedly worse than those in most mental institutions, and the risk of physical injury or sexual assault from other inmates is real. I make no apologies for the conditions of our nation's jails.[14] But this is no reason to continue to lock up harmless, noncriminal mental patients in mental hospitals. If our hesitation to subject the mentally disordered to jail is based on the conditions of our jails, we should be just as concerned about the impact of jail on those who are *not* mentally disturbed. Jails need major reform, but that hardly justifies using mental hospitals as backup jails. Again, confinement to a mental ward is also a form of arrest, and a particularly unfair one, since no criminal activity has taken place.

County jail inmates awaiting disposition of their cases need not be deprived of mental health services. Just as with the convicted felon in state prison, inmates in jail deserve treatment they can accept or reject. Abandoning forced treatment would improve treatment in jails, because inmates would no longer see the jail psychiatrist or psychologist as someone to be feared or manipulated. We need more, not fewer, voluntary treatment services in jails.[15] But we must offer services, not because we expect them to reduce crime or to reform criminals, but because mentally disturbed persons deserve real help, just as they deserve punishment if they commit crimes.

Finally, and most important, I favor jail over a locked mental ward for those relatively few mentally disturbed persons who commit crimes because mental wards cannot function as hospitals if they are serving as jails. By the use of locked wards we make mental hospitals into jails for all patients in the hope of saving a few from going to jail.

A Threat to Patients and Staff?

If a hospitalized mental patient disrupts ward routine or becomes assaultive or physically threatening, the behavior is almost inevitably labeled as "sick." The staff response is more drugs, by force. But this is the Catch-22: These disruptions may occur because the patient is frustrated and angry at being detained and forcibly drugged in the first place. Resistance to coercion is hardly a sign of mental disorder, yet resistance becomes a justification for more of the same treatment.

A patient's file often reports his or her "agitation," but this frequently is only a way for the ward personnel to describe attempts to resist medication or leave the hospital. The hospital usually wins the power struggle that ensues. Earlier ages used straitjackets, cold sheets, electroshock, and even lobotomy. Today we use "seclusion" rooms, leather "restraints," and drugs.

In these cases, the clearest indication that the person's behavior is a response to involuntary treatment rather than a sign of mental disorder is that no violence occurred until *after* the person was forcibly admitted to the hospital. A thirty-year-old man, for example, was handcuffed by police and taken to a local psychiatric ward. Why had this occurred? His parents had called the police because he was, in the words of the admitting psychiatrist, showing "grandiosity and inappropriate behavior." Although this was true, he had never lifted a finger to harm anyone or uttered a single threatening word. The police nevertheless removed him to the mental ward, where he refused medications. He was then wrestled to the floor, injected, and kept strapped in bed for several days. The psychiatrist wrote, "He could not be let out of restraints because of his unpredictable violent behavior." The message to the patient was clear: "You must do as we say, because if you resist, we will use whatever force is necessary."

What if society, through abolition of forced hospitalization and treatment, called a halt to this state of affairs? Far fewer patients would be disruptive or violent, for they would be given no reason to behave so, and we would be able to respond constructively to those few whose behavior was intolerable. Ward staff would tell the patient that his or her behavior was unacceptable and offer to help the person find a better way to express difficult feelings. If the behavior continued, the patient would be warned of possible discharge from the hospital. "We have many others," the ward staff would proclaim, "who are taking advantage of our help. We can't let you interfere with that." The repeatedly disruptive patient would simply be discharged. Physical assault would be dealt with as it is anywhere else: The police would be called and the person taken to jail.

What a turnabout! Imagine insisting, by force if necessary, that a mental patient *leave* the hospital rather than *stay* in the hospital. Since most violence in mental institutions results from the use of force *by the staff against the patients*, the truly free mental hospital would rarely be troubled by disruptive behavior.

Mental patients, even psychotic ones, do not lose control over every thought and every action. They would be able to refrain from unacceptable behavior if they knew that certain minimal standards of behavior were a requirement for receiving help. As things stand now, the patients know that no matter what they do, they will not be expelled from the hospital. Unlocking the doors of the mental ward and insisting on certain minimal standards of patient behavior as a requirement for receiving help would teach all of us—patients, families, professionals, and onlookers alike—that the behavior of the mentally disturbed person is a lot more responsible and responsive than we believe.

Interim Solutions

Until society is ready to abolish involuntary psychiatry, mental patients should have certain protections. Reforms of the past two decades have been too few and too timid. I recommend that the following steps be taken until we are ready to abolish coercive psychiatry. First, the legal protections of today's civil commitment laws must be enforced. Only a small percentage of those patients currently held and treated involuntarily actually meet the legal requirements for commitment. *Every* commitment should be reviewed by persons outside the treating facility. These investigators should have the power to initiate a hearing before a judge. The review should begin at the time the person is being *considered* for initial involuntary hospitalization. All persons found not to fit the legal criteria for commitment should be released.

Second, the use of sham "voluntary" admissions must stop. Each person being admitted to a mental hospital should be asked, by outside reviewers, if the consent is truly voluntary. Those found to have "signed in" under threat of formal involuntary admission must either be released or, if they in truth meet the legal criteria, be placed on formal involuntary status. Those transferred from pseudovoluntary status to openly involuntary status will be given *greater* legal protections against abuse than they now have. As long as involuntary treatment continues to be permitted by our laws, patients not free to leave a mental hospital are better protected if their lack of choice is clearly recognized by formal assignment to the involuntary category.

Third, a patient advocate should be available to every hospitalized patient, and advocates should never be in the employ of the hospital or mental health bureaucracy, as they are now. Law students or volunteer professionals might be suitable for this role, and would not unduly strain tax funds.

Fourth, civil commitment hearings should always be held in a court, never in a room at the hospital. The patient must have decent clothes to wear and must not be in a heavily drugged state. As things stand now, murderers come into court well dressed and clear-headed, while mental patients are led into a hearing room heavily drugged and disheveled. This is an affront to basic human dignity and biases the court.

The Dilemmas of Consent

If psychiatric treatment were always voluntary, the dilemmas of consent would be far fewer. No treatment would be given without the patient's approval. Until forced treatment is ended, interim changes should be made so that mental patients are treated more like other patients. Medical and surgical patients must give their consent before treatment may begin. This is because each person has the right to control his or her body and each person therefore has the right to exercise ultimate control over the doctor and the choice of treatment. When a patient consults a doctor, the doctor must describe the treatments available and the risks and benefits of each. Since the patient will bear the consequences of every choice, the patient must have the right of choice. In legal terms this means the consent must be both informed and free.

These ideals are, of course, not always followed. While doctors rarely try to coerce a patient into taking a treatment, they do often provide less than adequate information.[16] Several factors contribute to this. Doctors are busy, and may not give these matters a high priority. Many dislike being questioned about their judgments and recommendations. The patients, in turn, often want the doctor simply to tell them what to do, and prefer to take a passive role in treatment decisions. When this happens in medicine and surgery, it is because practice falls short of principle. In psychiatry, it is both practice and principle.

Mental patients are often denied the right to free and informed consent on the assumption that many of them have lost control of their minds and therefore do not have the capacity to exercise control over treatment decisions. Society says to the mental patient, "If we allow you in your irrational state to refuse treatments that might make you rational, you may never get well. Furthermore, if we accepted your refusal, we would then share in the responsibility for your continued irrationality."

This argument at first glance seems sound enough. Mental patients, particularly those placed on psychiatric wards, often are severely troubled; their disorders often do impair their judgments. They may engage in self-destructive behaviors, including the refusal of help that is sincerely offered.

Still, something is wrong. A major lesson from psychiatry's past (chapter 6) is that patients frequently turn out to be wiser in their refusals than the doctors in their insistence that a treatment go forward. As disordered as many patients may have been, they were not foolish enough to want lobotomies; yet fifty thousand were performed in the United States. Few asylum inmates willingly accepted the electroshock and insulin coma treatments of the 1940s and 1950s, but the doctors insisted. Most students of the development of psychiatry now agree that these treatments benefited the institutions, by making the inmates easier to manage, but damaged the patients. Even today's advocates of shock treatment, for example, agree that it was used in state asylums as a control device. Clearly, as bad as some patients may be at deciding what is best for them, psychiatrists may well be worse.

Why do patients' judgments turn out to be better than those of psychiatrists? Why have fully credentialed and often highly respected psychiatrists, with expert training and rational minds, defended treatments that only a few years later were seen to be highly abusive? Because psychiatrists, wittingly or unwittingly, frequently use their techniques as much for control as for treatment. Psychiatrists do not particularly enjoy controlling their patients. To argue that they do badly underestimates the real desire of most professionals to help their patients and fails to deal with the complexity of the problem. Rather, when psychiatrists serve more than one master, treatment easily becomes confused with control.

Psychiatrists are committed to helping, but through our laws and traditions we place unrealistic burdens on them. They are expected to change *behavior*, not just feelings. Often those most upset about the behavior are not the patients but relatives or other people. Without clearly recognizing the fact, the psychiatrist may be acting on behalf of third parties as much as on behalf of the patient.

How can these competing goals be resolved? By giving the patients the final say, we place responsibility on the only person who has the moral and ethical and medical right to it. Some will deny themselves help, to be sure, but far fewer than are now denied help by our insistence on involuntary treatment. For treatment is most often refused because of the power of psychiatry, not the disorder of the patient.

Given the present reliance on involuntary commitment, how can we best protect patients from abusive treatments? Are there means to give patients the final say about treatment, despite their not yet having the final say about hospitalization?

Respecting the Patient's Wishes

If a mental patient consents to a treatment, no one asks any questions. The patient is assumed to be competent to consent, and the consent is assumed to be free and informed. Whatever pressures may have been applied to gain this consent are simply ignored. No one asks, furthermore, whether the patient was given adequate information on which to base consent. Only if the patient refuses treatment are any questions asked. The person's competence to refuse may then be questioned. Mental patients, in other words, are generally considered competent to give consent, but incompetent to withhold it. This practice is exactly the opposite of how consent should be handled. *I propose that all mental patients be presumed competent to refuse any treatment. Refusal should never be overturned by a doctor or a court.*

Critics may respond by comparing the mental patient to the unconscious medical patient, and argue that this proposal would amount to leaving the person to die because he or she cannot consent to lifesaving treatment.[17] This, however, is a distortion of the true nature of mental disorders. Mental patients may have serious problems, but they are hardly unable to express their wishes. Unconscious patients, as well as the mentally retarded and very young children, are truly unable to comprehend treatment decisions. But mental patients know quite well how they feel about the effects of psychiatric treatments and are quite capable of accepting or rejecting a treatment. Very few are legally incompetent.

If a patient's refusal of treatment could not be overruled either by a treating psychiatrist or by a judge, mental patient advocates could devote their efforts to other problems and concentrate on reviewing situations where the patient has apparently *agreed* to a treatment. Advocates would check to see if the patient has been told about the risks of the treatment and if the patient is free from undue pressure to agree. Does the patient instead believe he or she must accept the treatment in order to avoid transfer to a state mental hospital? Has the psychiatrist told the patient he or she will have to go elsewhere for help if the treatment is refused? Such pressures are common on mental wards. Only when the review process found consent to treatment both informed and free would treatment proceed.

This review need not involve a court hearing, but the reviewers would be independent of the treating facility. The focus of the review would *not* be the patient's competence, as it is now, but the behavior of the doctor and the treating facility. Consent might be deemed invalid and treatment stopped, not because a patient's wishes could be invalidated, but because his or her apparent consent turned out to be ill informed or coerced. Psychiatry's record of past and current abuses mandates this approach.

When all this is said, however, it must be added once more that there is one step that can make these stringent measures unnecessary: the abolition of involuntary treatment. The extension to mental patients of what medical patients already have—final control over their treatments—is the best way to deal with the dilemmas of consent in psychiatry. Until then, the most vigilant protections will be necessary, and even these will fall short of what a free society owes to all its citizens.

A Free Market Mental Health System

Psychiatry monopolizes mental health care through its legal authority to treat patients involuntarily. Preferred treatment is also granted to psychiatry by government agencies and insurance companies, which pay the bills. Both of these advantages rest on the belief that the medical credentials of the psychiatrist justify the special powers and special financial arrangements. Granting psychiatry this level of influence has meant that a certain approach to mental health care has predominated. In order to best serve the mentally disturbed, we must offer more variety in treatment options. I am appalled that seriously disturbed persons have virtually no choice but to accept powerful mind-altering drugs in order to receive other kinds of help. I propose that we develop an alternative to the mental hospital.

A mental health facility should not be a medical facility. The mental hospital, as well as the mental ward of a general hospital, are enormously expensive because of their *medical* nature. This is wonderful for private mental hospitals and for psychiatrists' income but harmful to patients. Why? Medication is bound to be central to the treatment of a patient in a hospital. Other physical manipulations, like shock treatment, which only mask problems instead of helping the patient confront them, are also more likely in a hospital setting. The medical nature of a hospital also encourages persons with emotional problems to consider themselves "sick." It is then easier for them to wait for the experts to cure their problems. A hospital setting also encourages regressive behavior, because in a hospital patients are not expected to do much for themselves.

Judi Chamberlin, a former mental patient and now a leading advocate for alternative mental health care, has commented on the drawbacks of using a medical facility like a hospital to help persons who are emotionally distraught.

> Mental hospitals as they currently exist cannot provide this atmosphere of nurturance and growth. If the whole rhetoric of illness and pathology means anything, it means that parts of people's personalities are defective and diseased, fit only for medical tinkering.[18]

We need to develop a range of nonmedical alternative services in which psychiatry will not predominate over other legitimate mental health disciplines. The psychiatrist should play a minor role in mental health care because emotional disorders are not medical diseases. Nonmedical therapists and counselors could do a better job for less money. Psychiatrist Peter Breggin has noted, "At present the medical monopoly, supported by health-insurance programs, permits the enormous inflation of fees in a field in which many nonmedical therapists could compete at much lower rates." Breggin has also described, in terms consistent with my own thinking, his vision of "a haven" for mentally disturbed persons. He writes:

> In my ideal the most important service is the provision of a *safe space*—an environment that is comfortable, homelike, and secure, one in which the individual would feel able to rest, to think, or to socialize. Instead of walls being used to confine inmates, the walls of this haven would protect the clients from unwanted intrusions from friends, relatives, or authorities.

Persons in this place would, of course, be free to come and go. They would no longer need to fear psychiatry. With more alternatives to choose from, and with the final authority to decide which type of treatment is appealing, mentally disordered persons would finally enjoy the power and respect the rest of us take for granted. Our society owes this to mental patients. We owe it to ourselves.

CHAPTER 10

THE CRIME OF TREATMENT

The influence of psychiatry reaches into every corner of the life of a person who is mentally disturbed, but we could also say that psychiatry has the same pervasive influence for every person who faces confinement, including confinement in prison. Psychiatry has a tremendous impact on both the theory and practice of our prisons, but this impact has not been a useful one, either in the protection of society or in the rehabilitation of lawbreakers.[1]

The fundamental connection between psychiatry and prisons results from how we sentence a criminal offender. Well over a century ago reformers began to reason that the best way to reform a criminal was to consider illegal behavior a disease or disorder. Prison sentencing should focus on the individual prisoner's psychology as well as on the crime. Prisoners should be treated for their problems and held as long as, but no longer than, necessary.[2] The role of psychiatrists and other mental health professionals would be to carry out the treatment and inform parole officials when the prisoner was rehabilitated and no longer dangerous.

It sounded ideal, both for society and for those offenders willing to reform. Conservatives asked, "Why should society release the still-dangerous criminal after a fixed term, simply because he has done his time?" And liberals asked, "Why should a fully treated and reformed offender, no longer dangerous, be held years longer just to satisfy a fixed prison term?" But the sweet dream turned out to be a nightmare, as most commentators now recognize. To begin to understand why, let us look at one example in detail, one that illustrates clearly how psychiatry promotes injustice in our prisons.

The Case of Rodolfo Rodriguez

On June 20, 1952, twenty-six-year-old Rodolfo Rodriguez told a Los Angeles County Superior Court that he was guilty of fondling a six-year-old girl. According to court records,

> On the afternoon of April 20, 1952, [Rodriguez] and his wife were driving in their automobile when they saw six-year-old Sally roller skating. Petitioner stopped the car, got out, picked up the girl and put her on the front seat of the car next to his wife. They drove to a less public place where petitioner fondled the girl's private parts. Petitioner's wife, who was present throughout, repeatedly assured Sally that she would not be hurt. When curious citizens investigated the parked car, they found that the child's skirt was raised above her knees and that petitioner's trousers were unzipped. At the preliminary hearing the prosecution's expert medical witness testified that his examination showed no penetration of the sexual organs of the victim.[3]

Under California's system of indefinite, rather than fixed, sentencing, Rodriguez was given a term of one year to life in the state penitentiary. The date of release would be up to the parole board. The board, however, was in no hurry to release him. They knew he had been charged with sexual offenses on several previous occasions, sometimes involving children. They knew, moreover, that despite these previous charges, he had never been sent to prison. Instead, he had been committed to a mental hospital after criminal charges were dropped (an example of how reliance on the mental health system promotes criminal behavior, by excusing it). They knew finally that the last time this happened he had escaped from the mental institution. They had also recently received a letter from the district attorney asserting that Rodriguez "should never be released." Many parents in Rodriguez's neighborhood voiced the same sentiments.

For twenty-two years parole officials refused to release Rodriguez. Although he had never taken a life, he had been confined two or three times longer than are most convicted murderers. His case finally came to the attention of the San Francisco public interest law firm of Public Advocates. They filed a writ of habeas corpus on his behalf before the California Supreme Court, arguing that twenty-two years was too long a term for the crime he committed, and that the parole authorities showed every sign of keeping him behind bars for life. In addition, one of Rodriguez's attorneys called me early in January 1975 to ask if I would review the psychiatric reports and prepare an affidavit on my findings. I agreed. After I had read the material, it was clear that psychiatric reports were the major evidence being used to hold Rodriguez year after year.

At first prison psychiatrists considered him to have only the mildest of mental problems. He was diagnosed as having a "personality disorder," rather than a neurosis or schizophrenic psychosis; he was said to be making a "satisfactory institutional adjustment." Then, for two years, Rodriguez was diagnosed as having "schizophrenia." Whether he actually suffered a psychotic breakdown at that time was difficult to tell from his records. But even if this happened, what came next was crucial: He was diagnosed as having "schizophrenia in remission." This label was reapplied every year for the next twenty years. Regardless of how rational Rodriguez was said to be each year by psychiatrists, he was still "a schizophrenic."

As I reviewed his records, I also found something else. Three separate psychiatric reports—those of July 13, 1959, July 14, 1960, and September 11, 1961—were identical except for the date, which had been changed. Each year the psychiatrists had retyped the previous year's report, presenting it to the parole board as a new evaluation. And each year the parole board had accepted the "new" report as evidence of Rodriguez's current status.

By the time he had been incarcerated for ten years, Rodriguez felt he had paid his debt to society. His prison behavior had shown no disciplinary problems, and he consistently received good comments from work supervisors. After he told his counselor that he could not understand why he was being held so long, the counselor reported to the parole board: "Subject appears to have evaluated his present predicament as mere confinement. Little if any remission appears to have taken place regarding subject's emotional problems."

As I reviewed the parole board's yearly reports, I found that Rodriguez's feelings about "mere confinement," far from being a sign of mental illness, were quite justified. There was clear evidence that both the psychiatrists and the parole board intended to keep Rodriguez for life. The psychiatrists openly told the parole board that "he is a person who will probably need a lifetime in an institution." Their personal sensitivities came into play here: The psychiatric staff was angry at him because after years of group counseling in prison, Rodriguez refused to participate any further. They appeared to be punishing Rodriguez by calling this rebuff evidence of continuing mental disorder.

They also labeled Rodriguez's poor English as evidence of "psychotic thought fragmentation." They found it psychotic that he could not coolly and smoothly articulate his pent-up frustrations after so many years of lockup. Similarly, they linked his difficulty with reading—they called him "functionally illiterate"—to a supposed need for lifelong imprisonment. They had given him an IQ test years before, on which he had scored 68. This is "borderline mentally retarded," should one choose to place any faith in such tests. The test, which was given in English, never took into consideration that Rodriguez, a poor Mexican-American, had very limited skills in reading. His score said nothing about his true mental capacities, yet the psychiatrists considered it clear evidence that he was "defective."

Rodriguez rightly sensed something was going on behind the scenes when he called his stay "mere confinement." Indeed in their September 17, 1963, report the parole board bluntly called Rodriguez a "warehouse case," thereby admitting that in certain cases they ignore an inmate's "progress" or real psychological status; instead they make up their minds to store the person for life in prison. The yearly psychiatric reports were rituals, used to cover up the real intention of keeping Rodriguez in prison until he died.

Had his plight not been brought to the attention of influential lawyers, Rodriguez would still be a prisoner. Instead, California's Supreme Court heard his plea for release and ruled in his favor. They noted that

> his lack of "parole readiness" is not based on misconduct in prison but because the [parole board] cannot predict his future behavior, and because he is believed to lack ability to care for himself and to conform to parole requirements except in a structured living situation with supervision.[4]

Obviously talking about the psychiatric reports, the court then became more explicit.

> If petitioner is a "chronic schizophrenic," the basis for that diagnosis is not apparent in the records . . . the annual psychiatric evaluations in this file confirm that the condition has been "in remission" for the past twenty-two years. The conclusion of the Authority that his future conduct is "unpredictable," if based on that diagnosis, is questionable at best.[5]

Taking Another Look

The practice of giving indefinite sentences has turned prison terms into a very subjective matter. The date on which a prisoner is released depends as much upon guesses about whether the person is still dangerous as upon any fair legal guidelines based on the crime committed. An indefinite sentence is especially oppressive because it subjects *every* prisoner to the uncertainty and potential unfairness that results from rule-by-personal-opinion. If a prisoner serves as much time as the crime warrants, this is only a matter of chance.[6]

The attempt to make prisons into "reformatories" began in the early nineteenth century. Progressive thinkers said criminals should not simply be judged and punished. They should also be reformed.[7] Each era had its favorite theories about the "criminal mind" and how to remodel it. Mid-nineteenth-century reformers believed that corruption, drinking, prostitution, and general carousing of the cities pushed the "dangerous classes" to crime. The answer was a hearty dose of clean and orderly living—in prison. During their stay the deformed character of slum-dwelling criminals would be straightened, and they would finally become law-abiding citizens. By the end of the nineteenth century a strong medical focus (still with us today) had replaced the earlier emphasis on "moral degeneracy." Criminals were increasingly described as "sick" or "defective" rather than bad. From this it followed that like any decent hospital or clinic, the "reformatory" should treat its "patients" for as long as necessary.

This was a time of great discoveries in medicine, particularly in the control of contagious diseases. Should not crime also be considered a type of contagion? If so, are not the doctors of the mind the ones to cure criminality? As one textbook stated,

> The individualization of disease, in cause and in treatment, is the dominant truth in modern medi-

cal science. The same truth is now known about crime . . . the great truth of the present and the future, for criminal science, is the individualization of penal treatment—for that man and for the cause of that man's crime.[8]

Reformers convinced themselves that benevolent theories would be transformed into equally benevolent practices. A prisoner's treatment should be

varied according to his special need, which may, or may not, be painful in its operation . . . they will inflict no moment of unnecessary suffering; if they have to give any pain, there will be purpose in it, and a friendly purpose.[9]

My favorite quote from this period is the following. Convicts should be

banished to some kind of a colony or institution where they shall remain until definitely cured or transformed. If that be for life so be it. *It is not a punishment but a kindness* both to themselves and to society [emphasis added].[10]

Eventually the Freudian revolution prevailed, and psychoanalytic ideas became fashionable. By 1953 the leading textbook of criminology could claim that

if we are to develop a scientific philosophy of penal treatment compatible with the advances made by social and medical sciences during the past quarter century, *the concept of punishment must be completely dissipated.* If a criminal does what he must do in light of his background and his hereditary equipment, it is obviously both futile and unjust to punish him . . . it would be as foolish to punish him for having contracted tuberculosis [emphasis added].[11]

The criminal should instead be

> subjected to thoroughgoing examination of the
> psychopathic laboratory . . . with the development
> of methods for studying the physical and mental
> make-up of individuals, including intelligence test-
> ing, psychoanalysis, and the improved principles of
> psychiatry, behavioristic study has become to a
> large degree possible and profitable, and today as
> never before we are provided with the means for
> the understanding, explanation, and control of
> human behavior.[12]

By the 1960s the psychoanalytic mystique had begun
to fade and the behavior modifiers were popular. Psychologist James McConnell expressed the new hope in particularly stark form:

> The day has come when we can combine sensory
> deprivation with drugs, hypnosis and astute manip-
> ulation of reward and punishment to gain almost
> absolute control over an individual's behavior. It
> should be possible then to achieve a very rapid and
> highly effective type of positive brainwashing that
> would allow us to make dramatic changes in a
> person's behavior and personality. I foresee the day
> when we could convert the worst criminal in a
> matter of a few months—or perhaps even less time
> than that.[13]

A few of these programs were attempted, but they quickly
ran into strong opposition and were abandoned, though
not before things were done that should once again make
us leery of placing too much power in the hands of mental
health professionals.[14]

Anectine, for example, the same drug used to paralyze
the muscles during shock treatment, was for a while being
used on recalcitrant prisoners. Almost immediately after

the drug was injected into a prisoner, he would be unable to breathe. The frightening effect of this was precisely what the "treatment" was all about. It was considered "aversive conditioning." A prisoner who helped administer the treatment described it this way.

> The doctors drain Anectine from a vial while technicians wheel an oxygen tank closer. They will tell Harvey if he had behaved himself they wouldn't have to do this. The cotton ball will be cold on the tied vein, the needle inserted before he has time for a full breath or thought. Paralysis will sweep through him, pounding heart stilled, lungs unable to draw or burst, attempts at movement aborted. He will know he is dead as the doctors bend to softly warn, "Now, Harvey, you won't act up anymore will you? It just doesn't pay. You know better than that . . ." And before unconsciousness, before a blurred hand reaches for the tank, he'll revive, tingling with frightened life, no wiser from knowing the next dose will be larger.[15]

Facing Reality

By the 1970s prison reformers were finally recognizing that our century-long experiment with indefinite sentencing and prisoner rehabilitation was a failure. Studies showed that recidivism rates were not reduced by treatment programs.[16] The evidence indicated that neither parole officials nor prison psychiatrists knew when a prisoner was ready for release.[17]

The prisoners began to express themselves with an eloquence that came as a surprise to many, saying they would rather be considered "bad" than "mad."[18] They made it clear that they felt manipulated and degraded by therapy programs. Honest punishment was fine, they said, but not the humiliating punishment of playing the "therapy game."

Shortly after being sent to California's Folsom State Prison, Alfred Hassan wrote:

> If a man has done something so bad that we can't stand to look at him, then shoot him. But don't tamper with his soul. If he is a tyrant, then relieve him of his misery with a bullet in the brain. But don't whip his mind. Don't lie to him when he knows you are lying. Don't hand him that shit about rehabilitation . . . You can beat the flesh but it will soon become accustomed to the pain. But the mind is very, very tender. It can stand so much.[19]

When prisoners talked about the "lie" of rehabilitation, they were saying that they did not believe that the "experts" (psychiatrists, caseworkers, parole board members) were able to measure a convict's progress toward "rehabilitation." They considered the process worse than a sham—worse, because while the administrators and therapists claimed that indefinite sentences and group therapy sessions were tools of rehabilitation, the convict and his family knew they were really tools of manipulation. As Hassan wrote, "A prisoner has no idea at all when he will be released . . . He can only guess and this guessing game infuriates him."[20]

Hassan's wife suffered equally from the uncertainty.

> Each time I told my wife I had been denied parole she suffered tremendous pain. I remember the time . . . my wife wrote me a letter telling me she sensed (woman's intuition) that I was going to get a parole date. This made me feel very good and warm inside. But the roof, the world, fell in. I was denied parole! . . . the following week she came to visit me . . . I knew from the way she was looking that she expected me to run up to her and hug her and tell her that I would be home in a few weeks or a few months . . . I swallowed hard and broke

> the sad news . . . when she finally accepted the
> truth, it seemed like all the life was draining out of
> her plump face. Tears came to her eyes. I had never
> seen her look so sad. I felt like crying myself. I
> knew the pain and suffering she was going through.
> I was hard and calloused. But my sweet Mary was
> so tender and soft . . . From that point on, my wife
> was a different person. I think she lost all of her
> soul right there in that visiting yard. A year later
> she got sick and died of double pneumonia.[21]

Like most convicts, Hassan was not asking for sympathy
or denying responsibility for past crimes. He merely wanted
the benefit, both for himself and his family, of *knowing*
the extent of his punishment. As he said,

> Had I been given a parole date, I truly believe that
> my wife would be living today . . . Even if my wife
> knew that I was going to be in prison for ten or
> twenty years, knowing the exact date of my parole
> would have given her something concrete to look
> forward to. There wouldn't have been all the sad
> letters and disappointments.[22]

Over and over, interested outsiders hear the same refrain
from convicts. "Tell us our punishment," they say, "but
don't keep us dangling."

In today's prison, officials infinitely prefer running the
"time game"—that is, promising prisoners earlier release
dates in return for "good" behavior—to wielding old-
fashioned prison brutality. "A more sophisticated psychological brutality," writes a prisoner whose experience behind bars goes back to the Great Depression,

> has replaced the billy clubs and loaded canes of the
> former era. And it is my firm conviction, com-
> monly shared with others who have matriculated
> through the prison system, the sophisticated psy-

chological brutality . . . inflicts even greater damage
than the loaded canes of yesteryear.[23]

Yet another irony surrounds the role of psychiatry in
parole decisions: Real therapy in prison becomes nearly
impossible. Most convicts believe it is a grave mistake to
talk too frankly with any prison counselor. There is simply
no way of knowing how one's comments will be interpreted. The convict feels that "everything he says may be
used against him." Convicts are not told what the counselor puts in the evaluations sent to the parole board and
this only adds to their distrust. If a prisoner is told by
parole officials that he or she *must* engage in some form
of "treatment," this creates so much resentment and sus-
picion that the person is rarely willing to engage in genuine
attempts at personal reform with a prison therapist.

Convicts and an increasing number of reformers now
recognize that psychiatry's current role in our prisons,
especially as it relates to the indeterminate sentence, is not
only useless but harmful. A few states have legislated more
fixed sentences. Even in these states, however, legislators
have hedged their bets with psychiatry. Psychiatrists are
still asked to examine prisoners and tell parole boards if
they are dangerous. Prisoners are still forced to accept
unwanted psychiatric treatments.

The time has come for us to accept the truth of our
predicament. Psychiatry cannot protect us from harm, and
it cannot free us from our responsibilities as members of a
community and a larger society. The decisions we make on
how to treat confined persons must reflect our values and
our knowledge. Our sentencing laws must allow psychiatrists to offer help to prisoners who want help, but must
not allow psychiatric opinions to influence either the length
or the nature of a punishment handed down by a court.
Sentencing must be based on justice, not treatment, on
what a criminal has done, not on what we fear he or she

might do. We can implement these principles by making certain changes in our laws.

First, indefinite penalties must be replaced by definite penalties that are based, not on opinions of a criminal's "psyche," but on the seriousness of his or her crime. Second, state legislatures should fix sentences for specific categories of crimes, leaving judges only a slight amount of leeway at the time of conviction to pass a normal, mitigated, or aggravated sentence. Third, alternative penalties to prison sentences must be more thoroughly explored for nonviolent offenders. Fourth, convicted lawbreakers must be protected from involuntary psychiatric treatments. Fifth, parole surveillance should be abolished.

These recommendations reflect two assumptions: a person convicted of a crime is entitled to just punishment for that crime, and psychiatry is a healing art and ceases to heal if applied in any other manner.

In Praise of Punishment

Before discussing specific recommendations in detail, let me attempt to rescue the concept of criminal punishment from the rhetoric that has clouded our thinking for over a century. French sociologist Michel Foucault has written:

> In modern justice and on the part of those who dispense it there is a shame in punishing, which does not always preclude zeal. This sense of shame is constantly growing: The psychologists and the minor civil servants of moral orthopaedics proliferate on the wound it leaves.[24]

During the last one hundred and fifty years, the doctrine of *parens patriae* (the state as parent) has held that if treatment is good for almost everything, punishment is good for almost nothing. Throughout this book we have seen the unfortunate results of this thinking. The innocent (mental patients) are punished (involuntarily hospitalized and treated), while the guilty (criminals) are either excused or penalized with capriciousness rather than fairness. In the hope that we might begin to feel less of the shame that Foucault describes, and therefore do a better job of deciding who deserves punishment and how it should be administered, let me point out the virtues of punishment.[25]

First, punishment, once removed of its benevolent rhetoric, is honest. Society should say to the criminal, "You violated the law, and now you are being held accountable. We are not punishing you to make you a better person (though we hope you choose to learn from the consequences of your actions), but for our self-interest. We want to live in a society with rules, and rules become meaningless if there is no penalty for breaking them."

Second, punishment emphasizes justice and fairness. Based on overt acts that are measurable and definite, punishment can be graded according to the seriousness of the crime committed. Treatment cannot. Enforced therapy indeed takes no heed of ethical concepts like justice or fairness, because these concerns have no place in an individualized program of "help." Based on deviance as illness, individuals are "treated," not for what they have done, but for what they *are*.

Third, honest punishment is less destructive to the hearts and minds of convicts than is coercive treatment. By telling the convict when the punishment will end, we spare him or her the brutalizing effects of uncertainty. If individuals know they are being punished for what they did, not for who they are, they can maintain their dignity and personal integrity.[26]

Coercive "treatment," on the one hand, degrades and humiliates the person, because it scrutinizes every aspect of his or her being. It assaults the personality. And the convict must undergo unwanted treatments with a smile in order to convince the authorities that he or she is ready for release.

Honest punishment, on the other hand, recognizes the convict's right to remain "bad" if he or she so chooses.

The irony, however, is that when the convict has this choice, the person is more—not less—likely to seriously consider the need for personal reform. Instead of using his energy to resist the efforts of others to make him change, he is more likely to recognize the need to change himself. How do we know this? Because we all react to manipulations in the same way: None of us wants to change at someone else's command.[27]

Fourth, fixed punishments are less likely than indefinite punishments to encourage class and race injustice. The rhetoric of rehabilitation and the simultaneous renunciation of a punishment rationale have made it easier for an unfair criminal justice system—one that focuses most of its energy on the crimes of the poor while ignoring white-collar crime—to justify and even expand its unfairness. Honestly labeled punishments, on the other hand, encourage society to pay more attention to the necessary checks and balances on its power, by making people aware of a fair and definite standard whose application they can observe. When "therapy" is the mode of dealing with convicts, checks and balances are brushed off as a hindrance. When honest punishment is the mode, checks and balances are hailed as a constitutional necessity; courts are less likely to adopt a hands-off attitude. Since so much injustice permeates our society, the criminal justice system must take every opportunity to rid itself of unfairness.[28]

Just Penalties

Prisons are destructive institutions. They are intended to impose a painful (punishing) experience on the criminal and to control his or her behavior for a while. But they need massive reform so that they do not continue to be crippling agents that serve no useful purpose. The use of psychiatric theories and techniques in prisons has only magnified the problem. Society's "shame in punishing" indeed has not reduced unfairness. To the contrary, the denial of punishment as a legitimate response to crime has only made the poor and the powerless especially vulnerable. Fair and fixed penalties will obviously not solve our massive problems of social injustice, since these injustices result from economic and political inequalities in the wider society. But fair and fixed penalties would at least strip away the extra layer of injustice that results from the practice of indefinite criminal sentencing. I hope I have now given "punishment" some added respect. Let me examine now my five proposals for the development of a system of fair penalties.

Fixed Penalties—Let the Punishment Fit the Crime

Our criminal courts and prisons spend millions of dollars each year hiring mental health professionals to do probation evaluations, presentence reports, periodic treatment reviews, preparole reports, and postrelease evaluations. These professionals are, in Foucault's terms, our "minor civil servants of moral orthopaedics."

It is generally recognized that as a result of professional evaluations, the middle-class and white-collar person will more likely be treated leniently than the ghetto person. If Rodolfo Rodriguez had been Rudolph Roberts, he would probably not have spent twenty-two years in prison. Not all favoritism results from psychiatric evaluations; it may also result from biased behavior on the part of police and prosecutors. But the subjective element introduced by mental evaluations only increases the biases in our criminal justice system.

I believe we retain indefinite sentences out of fear. We fear that convicts will be released from prison while still dangerous, so we ask our experts to keep them until they are safe. There is much irony in this, for indeterminate sentences may allow murderers to leave prison in just a few years while confining nonviolent offenders for longer periods. This is a strange way to promote safety.

Sentencing as a Legislative Function

Not surprisingly, judges show the same variability of mood and temperament as the rest of us. Different judges may pass very different sentences for the same crime. Consequently, lawmakers have turned over part of the sentencing function to parole boards. But reliance on the parole system has not diminished sentencing inequities. Whether a sentence is set at trial by a judge, with the help of a mental health evaluation, or is determined much later by a parole board, also with the help of psychiatry, both focus on the wrong issue. Both pay attention to the individual's "mental health" rather than strictly to the crime.

State legislators, as the representatives of the people, should be the ones to codify punishments for the various classes of crime.[29] California's Uniform Determinate Sentencing Act of 1977 is an example of this approach. For each crime, the legislature identifies a median sentence. The judge must give this median sentence unless the facts of the individual case justify a mitigated or aggravated sentence.[30]

Sentences legislatively based on the nature of the crime rather than psychiatrically based on the nature of the criminal would thus be largely determined by the degree of harm done to society.[31] This mode of sentencing, based on justice instead of rehabilitation, would not only protect poor persons from being made into scapegoats by exaggerated attention to their "mental health." It would also prohibit white-collar and corporate crooks from unfairly benefiting from the same mental health examinations. The disrespect for law engendered when highly placed persons get probation while poor persons go to prison is not likely to promote law-abiding behavior. With legislatively fixed penalties, corporate criminals would more likely be punished as harshly as their crimes deserve, and people would gain more respect for the law.

None of this in any way implies a "lock 'em up and throw away the key" mentality. Rather it suggests that criminal penalties should be based on the values of the community, and codified by our representatives. If our values change, sentencing policies will also change. This is preferable to closed-door decisions by parole boards, on a case-by-case basis, where guesswork and prejudice may prevail.

Community-Based Penalties Should Be Expanded

Because prisons were supposed to do so much more than punish, we have relied on them too heavily. Convicted persons are, for the most part, either sent to prison or excused from any penalty whatever, except the requirement of periodically reporting to a probation officer. Thus we have a system of all or nothing. Programs that use community service as a punishment should be expanded, so that only violent offenders or those who use deadly weapons are sent to prison. The nonviolent offender would only go to prison if the person refused to cooperate with authorities while paying the penalty in the community.[32]

While society has the right to punish lawbreakers, we ought to do so in a way that does not punish ourselves. By sending even the nonviolent offender to prison, we not only spend too much of our money, we also make it less likely that the person will have a chance to rejoin the mainstream.

Separating Treatment from Punishment

Psychiatry should get out of the prison rehabilitation business. This does not mean that treatment services should not be available to criminals. As I have repeatedly stressed, abolition of forced treatment does not mean abolition of voluntary treatment. To the contrary, abolition of forced treatment, for convicts as much as for mental patients, will give psychiatric treatment a greater chance for success. The major reform necessary to separate treatment from punishment—abolishing indefinite sentences—would allow professionals to offer more, not less, help to convicts.

Prison psychiatrists would be free to devote their talents to helping prisoners with no requirement that they help maintain prison discipline or help determine parole dates. Trust, the essential ingredient of all therapies, would become possible, since the therapist would have no legal power either to force treatment on the convict or to influence the length of imprisonment. Mental health professionals might then also be more willing to work with prisoners.

Whether or not a convict elects to receive help would be a matter of indifference to prison officials, who would have only one responsibility: to punish the convict by confinement to prison for as long as the sentence dictates. If the convict is neither violent nor disruptive, the prison would be content to simply let the prisoner "do time." Difficult prisoners would be punished by loss of privileges or increased cell time, but no coercive psychiatric treatment (like drugs) could be used to control behavior.

Prison therapy is generally mistrusted by convicts.[33] This would change once the therapist's legal power to enforce treatment and to influence release dates was ended. As one former prisoner told me, "Lots of guys inside [prison] would accept help if prison officials stopped playing all the games with a parole date."

Abolishing Parole Surveillance

If all criminals sent to prison received fixed terms, parole would cease to exist. Criminals would not weep over this, for even the released prisoner may be subjected to years of surveillance and humiliating restrictions. Currently a person can be ordered not to leave the county of residence without permission, not to associate with other ex-convicts, and not to have a "common-law relationship." These absurd regulations are routinely ignored by former prisoners, and even by parole officers. Nonetheless, they may be invoked at the parole agent's discretion, and this possibility alone adds resentment and anxiety to the difficult problems already facing the parolee.

Parole is often used to force the released person to undergo mandatory psychiatric therapy, including the use of powerful mind-altering drugs. In this way therapy becomes a vehicle for maintaining control after release. If forced treatment and surveillance could be shown to reduce crime, these practices might be defensible, but research has not been able to find the presumed connection.[34] We do, however, spend a lot of money on these activities.

The abolition of parole would not, I hasten to add, mean an abolition of voluntary postrelease services, such as assistance with job placement or housing.[35] Ex-offenders, I believe, would more readily accept, and thus better utilize, voluntary services than the mandatory surveillance of parole.

In the fixing of criminal penalties, psychiatry can serve no useful role. Society's persistent attempt to give it a role has, in fact, merely added to the injustice of our criminal justice system while keeping psychiatry from its legitimate role—offering voluntary therapy to those prisoners who want it.

If society stopped expecting psychiatrists and related professionals to rehabilitate criminals, and thereby reduce crime, we might have a better chance of promoting public safety in other ways. Social reform, not individual psychological reform, is the key to reducing crime and violence.

CHAPTER 11

CHILDREN AND THE DOUBLE STANDARD OF JUSTICE

The confusion in our society between what is "help" and what is "punishment'" extends into the agencies and institutions set up to help needy children, on the one hand, or control delinquent children, on the other hand.

According to the philosophy of our juvenile justice system, everything is done for the good of the child, to help, never to punish. Judges do not oversee trials; instead "referees" conduct hearings. Guilt is not proclaimed; a "finding" is announced. Children locked up in a juvenile facility are not prisoners but "wards." The confinement is considered "care and treatment," rather than punishment.[1]

Others have written the history of the juvenile court movement.[2] I will only note here that the same benevolent rhetoric we have examined in the history of prisons led in the early years of the twentieth century to the establishment of special juvenile court proceedings. Those who have studied this development generally agree that the informality of the new juvenile court, which was supposed to protect the child from the harshness of the adult criminal justice system, has led to even greater injustice.[3] The President's Crime Commission stated in its 1967 report, "The great hopes originally held for the juvenile court have not been fulfilled."[4]

Punishing the Harmless Girl

The juvenile justice system is especially harsh on girls. Consider, for example, what happened to jazz singer Billie

Holiday. Born in 1915, she was raped at the age of ten by a neighbor. She later said, in *Lady Sings the Blues:*

> Instead of treating me and Mom like somebody who called the cops for help, they treated me like I killed somebody. They wouldn't let my mother take me home . . . they threw me into a cell. My mother cried and screamed and pleaded but they just put her out of the jailhouse and turned me over to a fat white matron . . . After a couple of days in a cell, they dragged me into court. Mr. Dick got sentenced to five years. They sentenced me to a Catholic institution.[5]

Under the juvenile court system, a child like Billie was not supposed to need any due-process legal protections. The judge, like a good father, would look after the child's best interests. She may have felt she was "sentenced" to the institution, but the juvenile court authorities believed they were providing her "protection."

Who was right? Here is how she described part of her stay at the institution. She had broken a rule and was being punished.

> They wouldn't let me sleep in the dormitories with the other girls. Another girl had died and they had her laid out in the front room. And for punishment they locked me in the room with her for the night . . . I couldn't stand dead people ever since my great-grandmother had died holding me in her arms. I couldn't sleep. I couldn't stand it. I screamed and banged at the door so, I kept the whole joint from sleeping. I hammered on the door until my hands were bloody.

To this very day, a girl who has committed no crime can be caught in the juvenile court network and saddled with the "state as parent." With relatively recent court decisions, beginning with the U.S. Supreme Court's 1967 ruling in

In re Gault that children needed greater legal protections in court, intrusions probably happen less often now than in the past.[6] But because the juvenile court system continues to be based almost entirely on the theory of kindly state intervention, justice may take a back seat to other considerations.

Lockup for one year, for example, might seem a harsh penalty for truancy, but that was the sentence for a fourteen-year-old girl I'll call Linda. Truancy, like running away from home or being "beyond parental control," is a "status offense," which means that the act is not a crime for adults, only for children. The "status" of being a child makes the behavior illegal.[7] For her behavior, Linda was sent to an institution where virtually all of the girls were guilty of status offenses. In Linda's case, she had started cutting school as a protest against her mother's working at night. There was no father in the home, and her mother felt she had to take an evening job as a cocktail waitress. After Linda had run away a number of times, her mother followed through on her threat to call the juvenile probation department. Initially taken to juvenile hall, Linda was eventually placed in a detention facility which though newly constructed and pleasant appearing nonetheless functioned as a minimum security prison. After a couple of months, both Linda and her mother had decided the "treatment was worse than the disease," and wanted to be reunited at home. By this time the staff had worked out a "treatment plan," which had a life of its own. Linda should stay until she had made up her lost school credits, they said, regardless of what she and her mother now wanted.

At the request of Linda's public defender, I reviewed her case. I talked extensively with the superintendent, who made it abundantly clear that she was the head of a *school*, not a prison, one functioning largely as a backup for the county truant officer. The county was quite prepared to lock up a child, perhaps for a year or even longer, if that was the only way to keep the youngster in the classroom. School credits must be earned before a return home would be possible.

Even though Linda's mother had now quit her night job, and was in a better position to supervise her, the county probation department was prepared to fight any possible release. Only when Linda's public defender and I sat in the juvenile court hearing room, ready to argue that continued confinement was only creating new problems, did the superintendent finally relent and agree to let Linda return to her mother's home. This was fifty years after Billie Holiday was taken from her home and her mother for "her own protection." Separated by half a century, a poor black girl and a working-class white girl had been locked up, not because either was guilty of any crime, but because each supposedly needed "supervision." In each child's case, the juvenile court's response only compounded the problem.[8]

Sociologist Celeste McLeod has studied such unfairness in our treatment of children. As she points out, the criminal sometimes goes free while the victim is locked up. Seventeen-year-old Mia, McLeod tells us, was living with her boyfriend. Her parents had given their consent. When she was "kidnapped and raped by another man . . . she reported it to the police." Because Mia was still a minor and living with a man out of wedlock, the police "arrested her as a runaway and shipped her off to juvenile hall instead of going after the rapist."[9]

Altogether, more than six hundred thousand children are arrested each year for acts that would not warrant arrest of an adult.[10] Most are girls who are officially deemed to be a "child (minor, person) in need of supervision." How many are held in some type of institution? According to Aryeh Neier, former executive director of the American Civil Liberties Union, "about 85,000 children a year are sent to long-term 'correctional' institutions. Of these children, twenty-three percent of the boys and seventy percent of the girls are found guilty of offenses that would not be crimes if committed by adults."[11]

It is no coincidence that my examples involve young women. These cases reflect a national pattern, in which girls guilty of noncriminal status offenses—running away, truancy, "incorrigibility"—are more likely to be locked up than boys found guilty of serious, and sometimes violent, crimes.[12] Indeed three-fourths of the girls in juvenile institutions are guilty of status offenses, whereas boys tend to be taken to court, not necessarily locked up, for crimes like burglary, robbery, or worse.[13] The final unfairness is that once detained, girls are incarcerated longer than boys. As Charles Silberman, in *Criminal Violence, Criminal Justice*, has said,

> Juvenile Court judges are the prisoners of their own rhetoric. In their desire to "help" troubled youngsters, they spend the bulk of their time on juveniles charged with offenses such as "incorrigibility," truancy, running away from home, and other behaviors that do not involve any direct threat to public safety. These "status offenses" . . . account for at least half, and perhaps as much as two thirds, of juvenile court time. As a result, little time or energy is left to deal with those juveniles who commit serious crimes.[14]

Why are girls punished more severely for noncrimes than are boys for dangerous crimes? The answer lies in the fact that the juvenile court system denies punishing anyone for anything. According to juvenile court philosophy, the child coming under its control—whether a murderer or a runaway—is *not* being punished, but protected and treated for the psychiatric disorder that is causing the behavior. What this jargon really means is that society is more offended by a girl on the loose than by a boy on a rampage.

Our sexual prejudices make us treat girls more protectively, which means more strictly or harshly. As one researcher has put it, "While most young women in the court were charged with status offenses, these were simply buffer charges to mask concern for sexual behavior."[15] Both the adolescent girl's family and the court feel they must place her in some protected setting to make sure she won't end up on the streets. Because it is often the parents who initiate state intervention, the girl has no one (except perhaps an overburdened public defender) to help her argue that incarceration is not the answer.[16] The juvenile court judge, faced with this pressure from the family, and instructed by a juvenile court philosophy that tells him to intervene in the name of "help," all too often feels obligated to order the girl placed in an institution.

When law professor Richard Chused studied the day-to-day workings of the juvenile court in three New Jersey counties, he saw these forces at work. "Juvenile status offenders were more likely to be female than were other types of offenders, and females were more likely to be detained than males." "Parents," Chused also found, "were not willing to come forward to assume custody of status offenders as often as in other cases."[17] Girls, finally, were often held in custody,

> as a device to deal with family disputes and other minor cases in a quick, decisive, and probably illegal, fashion. Females are more likely to be charged with offenses relating to sexual behavior than males and . . . such offenses may be treated severely by the judicial process.[18]

Does intervention actually help the young women who come before the juvenile court? In some cases it does, but in many cases it emphatically does not. Consider, for example, the findings of Meda Chesney-Lind. "Young women 'on the run,'" she writes, from homes characterized by sexual abuse and parental neglect are forced, by the very statutes designed to protect them, into the life of an escaped convict. Unable to enroll in school or take a straight job to support themselves because they fear detection, young female runaways are forced into the streets. Here they engage in panhandling, petty theft, and occasional prostitution in order to survive.[19]

To this perceptive analysis, I want to add a question. If a girl is beaten or killed while "hustling," is it an exaggeration to say that our present juvenile court system is an accessory to the crime?

The juvenile court functions more to reinforce parental wishes and societal prejudices than to offer either fairness or genuine help to the young women in need. Youngsters who are incarcerated and often unwillingly subjected to the state's "help" may be compared with mental patients who are locked up and treated against their will. In both cases, the innocent are punished.

Getting Away with Murder

The juvenile court system is also frequently unjust with boys, but in quite different ways. Young criminals, sometimes guilty of vicious crimes of violence, are often treated too leniently. Recently I asked a San Francisco district attorney assigned to a juvenile court to describe the usual pattern of dealing with the youthful male offender. His comments reflect a prosecutor's perspective, but they are nonetheless instructive. "Typically we set a kid up," he said. "What does that mean?" I asked. He replied,

Take a twelve-year-old who steals a bicycle. Nothing much is done and soon he's had four or five more thefts that are handled by the police as "kiss-

offs." By the sixth offense, bigger by this time, he's
handled informally by the probation department
without going to court. At fifteen he gets caught
for burglary. The referee [judge] sees that this is
his first time in court and places him on probation.
By the time he's sixteen or seventeen he's ready for
the heavy stuff, and no amount of talk is going to
convince him that he has much to lose if he gets
caught.[20]

I vividly recall a seventeen-year-old, after being arrested for
burglary, telling me, "I know I have to stop this because
when I'm eighteen they'll get tougher." Young offenders
can have no respect for an adult world that is too hesitant,
guilty, and hypocritical to punish them openly and honestly for criminal activity.

Writer Nicholas Pileggi in *New York* magazine presents
a striking example of how the juvenile justice system may
teach youngsters that crime pays. He begins the story on
February 23, 1977.

At 1:15 A.M., a yellow checker taxicab pulled up
to the tenement. The youngster inside the cab was
even smaller than his friends waiting outside. The
driver, a 26-year-old Brooklyn college student, began to automatically roll up his half-closed window.
The glass pane was about three inches from closing
shut when a shot rang out. The driver slumped
forward, lifeless, a bullet hole in his left temple.

The youngsters immediately tried opening the
driver's door, but it had been locked. They ran
around to the other side. Locked. One of them
jumped into the rear of the cab and tried sliding
open the partition separating the driver from the
passengers. They tried wedging their arms through
the partially opened window, but that didn't work
either.

Suddenly one of the trio ran part of the way down the block and returned, half carrying a ten-year-old boy whose arm was thin enough to fit through the narrow window opening. It was the ten-year-old who unlocked the cab. Once inside the youngsters rifled through the dead man's clothing and took $60 from his wallet. They were about to run off when one of the three remembered the driver's radio. He ran back to the cab. The radio was covered with blood. He took it anyway.[21]

Grisly as all this may be, events leading up to this murder are even more shocking. "Before George Adorno had reached his sixteenth birthday," Pileggi tells us, "he had admitted committing two homicides, having been in robberies involving two more killings, and having taken part in innumerable nonfatal robberies (about 40 taxicab stickups alone), some burglaries, and even an arson."

Standing barely over five feet tall and weighing no more than 120 pounds, George Adorno was, along with his friends, a powerful and feared element in his Harlem community. He was "part of a loosely organized neighborhood band of about a dozen teenage purse-snatchers, street muggers, armed holdup men, and killers. Robbing was what they did on a daily basis." Guns were easily rented from neighborhood contacts, for three to ten dollars per day. Local police estimated that Adorno's friends had been arrested over one hundred times, but added that "for every arrest, there are at least ten or even twenty street muggings or stickups committed."

Taxi drivers were a favorite target, since they always had plenty of money, more than enough to keep the boys well supplied with "junk food, kung fu films, and pinball" until they were ready for their next job. A typical taxicab robbery went like this.

One of them [would] approach the driver from the passenger's side while the cab is stopped for a light. While the first youth asks the driver about being taken to some address or other and the driver's attention is momentarily diverted, the other youngsters gather around the driver's window. One of the youngsters always has the gun and only rarely does the driver resist.[22]

Why, despite his previous rampages, was George Adorno free to roam the streets that night in February 1977 when Steven Robinson, the cab driver, was murdered? The answer to that question can teach us a lot about our juvenile justice system and its confused thinking about crime and punishment.

Since the age of twelve, young George had been the subject of many warrants for arrest. None of these warrants, however, had ever resulted in an actual arrest. Why? Because the Manhattan family court simply didn't have a warrant officer who could drive to George's home and take him into custody. Finally, after innumerable armed robberies and other crimes, George was placed in a juvenile detention facility. After three months he was given a pass to go home for several days; while back in the neighborhood he was arrested for another robbery. Since neither the police nor the court had been informed of George's placement; they did not know he was on a pass. Released shortly after his arrest, George simply returned from his pass with "no one the wiser." A week later he was given another pass, and was again arrested for robbery. Just as before, he was released by the juvenile court in time to return from his pass, and the institution still knew nothing of what he was doing on his weekend passes. Neither the police (on weekends) nor the detention facility (during the week) knew what George was doing when he left them. Throughout his "sentence," in fact, George continued his crime spree on his weekend passes. Whenever the police went looking for George, they could not find him because he had the perfect hiding place—the juvenile prison. As a result of family court policy, no one—not even the police—was allowed to know of George's whereabouts.

George was released on July 19, 1974. During the next four months four persons were killed and George later admitted to being involved in each instance. The first killing took place the very day he was released.

> He was walking along Lexington Avenue near 117th Street when he ran into two friends. One, a fourteen-year-old, was carrying a silver-plated .45 automatic. The other, who was fifteen, had a hunting rifle. The pair, Adorno said, told him they were on their way to stick up a local pawnshop owner. When they got to the location, Adorno said, the other two went inside while he waited across the street. He said he was not acting as a lookout but just wanted to see how they were going to do it. In a few minutes, Adorno heard some shots and saw the boys running out of the pawnshop with rings and gold medallion chains streaming through their fingers. The pawnshop owner was killed in the stickup.[23]

The next murder took place less than a month later. Adorno and five of his friends wanted a car. It was the early morning hours of August 18, 1974, when the group ran into a parking garage. A shot rang out and the parking attendant fell dead. Adorno claimed he was not the one who fired the gun.

Death came to their next victim just three weeks later, on September 7. This time Adorno left no doubt about what happened. As Nicholas Pileggi tells us,

> Adorno and two other pals were walking toward Eighth Avenue looking for a taxicab driver to stick

up. One of the boys went to the window opposite the driver and asked to be taken to 110th and Lenox. Meanwhile George walked up to the driver's window and saw that the man had some folded bills in his shirt pocket. George never hesitated. He simply put his hand in the cabdriver's shirt pocket and began to remove the money.[24]

When the driver resisted, George fired a bullet into his head. As he said, "He grabbed my hand . . . so I just shot him. I just went pop."

George was still roaming the streets five weeks later, even though the police and the courts knew which group of boys was involved in this murder. Adorno denied that he fired the fatal shot, but fourteen-year-old Michael Hurd was talking with the police. Then,

On October 24, five weeks after the cabdriver killing, George, T-boy, and Ray were shooting pigeons on a rooftop at 116th Street when they saw Mushmouth [Hurd] on the street below. The rifle, which belonged to Ray, had a scope. George said he took the rifle from Ray, aimed at Mushmouth's head and fired. Mushmouth died instantly.[25]

Four days later, George was questioned by authorities about the September 7 slaying of the taxi driver. Still just fifteen, the law required that a parent or legal guardian be present during the questioning. His father hadn't been around for years and his mother was in Puerto Rico at the time. His eighteen-year-old sister, who according to the district attorney was the most stable person in George's family, was called in to witness the questioning. Nonetheless, homicide charges against Adorno were later dismissed by family court judge Shirley Wohl Kran because George's mother was not present during the questioning.

Three weeks later, on January 20, 1975, a warrant for George's arrest was issued for a number of armed robbery charges. He was not actually apprehended until February 7th, even though he lived at home the entire time. When he was finally taken in, he had on his person a loaded .38 caliber pistol and seven envelopes of cocaine.

Finally, having reached age sixteen, George Adorno was locked up for armed robbery, and held until shortly after his eighteenth birthday. Then, only a few weeks after his release, George Adorno gunned down twenty-six-year-old Steven Robinson as he sat in his cab. George was charged with murder.

One of George's accomplices was still fifteen, and was sent to family court. Referred for psychiatric examination, the young man simply walked out of the unguarded clinic when the doctors were through with him. He went home, and it wasn't until a week later that authorities went to retrieve him. They found him dancing at the local community center.

George Adorno's case is not typical, but it illustrates the need for a major overhaul in our approach to violent juvenile crime. Further, the confusion between what is "help" and what is "punishment" continues into our juvenile "reformatories" and "training schools." Mental health professionals in these institutions are saddled with the same impossible mandate as those working in adult prisons: Rehabilitate inmates, whether or not they want to be rehabilitated. The results are no more successful than in adult prisons; sometimes the results are tragic.

The Suicide of Joe Grayson

A boy I'll call Joe Grayson was dead at seventeen by his own hand, and the state of California wanted to know why. Why had a boy being treated at one of the state's top treatment centers for juvenile offenders hanged himself in his cell? Joe's suicide clearly indicated that something was wrong at the Intensive Treatment Unit (ITU) outside Sacramento.

Joe's death was not the only troubling event: Lawyers representing many of the ITU's youthful offenders charged that numerous serious abuses were being carried out in the name of treatment. Faced with these charges, the California Youth Authority (CYA), in the summer of 1975, asked me to investigate not only Grayson's suicide but also the other inmates' allegations. Along with a lawyer, two social workers, and another psychiatrist, I began to investigate the charges.

The young men housed at the ITU were all guilty of serious crimes, many involving violence. Nonetheless, juvenile court rhetoric stated that they had been "committed" not for punishment but for "care and treatment." The "wards," as the young men were called, knew perfectly well, however, that they had been sentenced to prison. Within California's system of institutions for the most antisocial youth, the ITU was considered a model program, using the latest techniques of behavior modification and transactional analysis (TA). Subjective Freudian interpretations were definitely out of favor. Instead, the "ward" would "graduate" from the program (be released) only after he earned points by acting commendably and participating in the program.

The ITU's therapy program was divided into three "phases." As the ward moved into each level, he gradually won increasing privileges. Many of the boys refused to participate in this form of therapy. To force compliance, the administration resorted to harsh measures. That at least is what the young inmates' lawyers were claiming. They charged that the ITU was threatening to transfer wards to California's scariest adult prisons if the boys did not take part in the treatment programs. In addition, lockups lasting twenty-four hours were allegedly imposed "for the offense of refusing to attend group therapy." To illustrate their concerns, the lawyers reported an incident in which

a ward who closed his eyes during group . . . was told to go to his room. He asked if there was a written rule that wards couldn't close their eyes during group. He again was told to go to his room. When he refused, he was chained up, maced, sedated by drugs, and then locked in his room for seventy-two hours.

The lawyers also charged that the ITU was using inmates to punish and control others. Finally, the lawyers asserted that the treatment program itself was "psychologically brutal and primitive," because the inmates were forced to participate in order to qualify for parole. This is precisely what adult prisoners face under indeterminate sentencing.

When the five-member task force met for the first time, I was asked to take special responsibility for looking into the suicide of Joe Grayson. As I conducted my interviews with the ITU staff and inmates and reviewed Joe's file, I learned about his frustrations at not being able to move from Phase I to Phase II. He hadn't, in fact, wanted to go to the ITU in the first place, preferring his former program where vocational activities were emphasized. Within weeks of his arrival, Joe had tried to escape. His punishment was fifteen days of round-the-clock restriction to his "room," a cell with a solid door and a peephole.

Staff members noticed that he became "decidedly negative" during this period. Even when the fifteen-day punishment was over, his mood stayed low. Several young inmates told me that "Joe had been asking to get out of the program, but Edison [the director] said no."* Joe also told them that "if he couldn't get out by running, he would get out by pine box. He didn't see how he could make it through the program. He just didn't want to do it."

What was it that Joe Grayson didn't want to do, so much so that he was willing to die instead? Play the game of prison therapy: talk about himself. "He sometimes

---

*All names have been changed.

refused to even go to the group therapy," several of his friends told me. He was particularly despondent because, as they said, "he couldn't get out of the ITU until he talked about himself, but he refused to talk." The only way to get through Phases I, II, and III and get a recommendation for parole, I learned from ITU staff, was to participate in the "TA games," which were so important in the group sessions. As one of Joe's closest friends told me, "He just didn't want to do it, he didn't like the TA. The last week he was in his room all the time, for refusing to participate. He felt he would never get out of here. I don't think this would have happened at another program." A staff member agreed: "He was very quiet the week before it happened. He told me he didn't think he'd ever get out of here."

When his body was found hanging from a light fixture on April 14, 1975, a note was also found in his cell. "I am locked up," he had written, "because I was feeling pretty bad over some broad, and when they came to get me for group [therapy] I told them to beat it."

I was not prepared to say in my report to the Youth Authority that forced therapy "caused" Joe Grayson's suicide, but I did conclude that it was an aggravating factor that not only failed to help but probably added to the pressures leading to the suicide.

Games Prisons Play

When I read some of the official documents describing the ITU treatment program, I could easily understand why the young prisoners felt trapped. Like the behavior modification programs in adult prisons, ITU's program said, "Talk, or else. No talk, no parole." A new inmate at ITU had to negotiate a "contract" with the staff. These negotiations, of course, were patently unfair. The prison had all the power; the prisoner had none. Nonetheless, promises were made, in which the ITU agreed to recommend the youth for parole if he, in turn, would keep out of trouble *and* be a good patient in the group therapy sessions. As the program administrators said, "If you are meeting your goals in counseling . . . your counselor will recommend you to Phase II."

Phase II brought the expected increase in privileges, like "free access to your room," "late stay-ups," and "day passes with your family." Those who, like Joe Grayson, were simply not willing to talk about personal feelings would languish in Phase I as long as their stubborn refusal persisted. Parole, of course, was out of the question for anyone still in Phase I.

As the week progressed, our task force became convinced that the charges brought by the young prisoners and their lawyers were justified. Because three of the five members were employees of the CYA, there was intense pressure to present our findings in a moderate tone. Nonetheless, we concluded that "wards are coerced to participate in the treatment program . . . in order to earn a referral to parole." We further found that the ITU staff even considered lockup to be part of the treatment program. We wrote:

> The staff made little or no distinction between treatment and punishment . . . Lockups for violations of the rules are . . . part of the treatment . . . There were a great number of cases that involved what appeared to be rather minor violations, such as making too much noise in the day room, horseplay, asking to leave group, being late to breakfast or school, walking on the grass, etc. for which 24-hour lockup was the solution . . . punishment has taken place under the guise of treatment.

Regarding the "phase system" of the ITU, we wrote that while "ITU staff view the phase system as a treatment tool, in essence and practice the major reason for the phase system is management, control, motivational purposes and only incidentally as treatment." Finally, particularly disturbing was that some prisoners were being used to control other prisoners, as inmates had alleged. Those who had made it to Phase III helped run the program, recommended lockup, carried keys, and even made recommendations on whether or not a youth would be promoted from Phase I to Phase II.

Was It Brainwashing?

The lawyers representing the inmates at ITU went even further in their charges. They alleged that "forced confessions" (group therapy), twenty-four-hour lockup for failure to participate, and the use of co-opted prisoners to browbeat new prisoners added up to "brainwashing" of the sort used by the North Korean and Chinese communists against our soldiers during the Korean War of 1950–1953. As the only member of the task force who had previously studied the subject of "brainwashing" or "coercive persuasion," I was again asked by the others to write a supplemental report on this question. Was the ITU using brainwashing?

Based on what I had seen during our week-long investigation, I could indeed see little distinction between the ITU's "treatment" program and what had been done in Korea. In both, the essential ingredient of *captivity* was present. In both, as I wrote in my report, the prisoner knew "that if he will show signs of incorporating new ways of thinking and feeling, life will be made more pleasant for him." In both, "the group is often the vehicle" for coercive persuasion. In both, "the use of other captives for the administration of thought reform is an inherent part of the effort." In both, favored prisoners

> have a great deal of investment in getting their new
> recruits to show signs of real change, because these
> upper class captives can only maintain their privi-
> leged status if they demonstrate that, in addition

to their own thought reform, they are also effective in causing thought reform in the new recruits.

I also pointed to one ironic feature, which made the use of "brainwashing" on Americans by Americans even more demeaning than what had been done to Americans by Koreans. In Korea, those who most firmly resisted the pressures would later be cited by America for their commendable behavior, whereas in American prisons those who refused to cooperate were considered "resistant to treatment."

Within days after we submitted our report to the CYA, we were told that its contents should be considered confidential. The CYA appeared anxious to file the report on a dusty shelf, with only a promise that whatever excesses we found at the ITU would be remedied. Their response was hardly surprising, since those in charge of programs for juvenile offenders are not given a clear and honest mandate from society. Society in truth turns over youngsters for punishment, control, and management, but still pretends (even more so than with adults) that treatment, and treatment alone, is the purpose of confinement. It is not surprising, therefore, that programs like the ITU have never been shown to make a lasting impact on youthful offenders.

Justice for Children

Like adults, children who have committed no crimes deserve to be helped, free of punishing therapeutic controls, and children who have committed crimes deserve to be punished with honesty and justice. Our present juvenile court system does not make this distinction. Rather it just as often punishes a child (usually a girl) who has committed no crime as it excuses a child (usually a boy) who has committed one or more crimes. This injustice occurs because society expects a single juvenile court system to accomplish contradictory objectives: to help some of its clients and to control others.

Charles Silberman, in *Criminal Violence, Criminal Justice*, has written:

> Ambivalence is built into the very marrow of the juvenile court, which is expected both to nurture and to protect the young against older members of society, and to protect society against the misbehaving young.[26]

When the same agency is told to control vicious criminals, on the one hand, and to offer loving care and protection to abandoned, mistreated, or needy children on the other, it gets its goals mixed up. After eighty-five years, the juvenile court system seldom accomplishes either goal.

The solution is to develop two independent juvenile court systems: one to help children in need, and another to control and punish young criminals. In this way children and society would be better served. The helping system would never punish noncriminal behavior, but would offer the child ways to protect his or her interests. The punishment system, on the other hand, would serve as a criminal justice system. It would be in the business of control and punishment, and would make no apologies for this.

Helping the Innocent Child

Here, the *parens patriae* doctrine would finally find a legitimate home, for some children do need substitute parents. The physically or sexually abused child does require protection. The neglected child does have a right to decent care. Since children cannot protect themselves, state intervention is appropriate.

We must distinguish at this point between genuinely benevolent intervention and using psychiatrists' opinions to determine children's needs. We should not call in psychiatrists, I believe, because delicate decisions about child custody and protection require informed opinions but not "expert" opinions. A case may, in other words, require investigations but not "examinations." *I recommend that we never solicit psychiatric evaluations in deciding issues of child custody and protection.*[27]

Because psychiatric examinations are so unreliable and not infrequently downright foolish, they may hinder rather than promote the best interests of a child. Consider the following. A man I'll call Joe Robinson had two sons by a previous marriage. His children, four-year-old George and three-year-old Randy, were living with their mother and her boyfriend, Chris, when a tragic event occurred. The children were watching television while their mother was napping. Chris was away. George had noticed Chris's gun before and now he saw it on the floor by the couch. His sleeping mother was jolted awake by the sound of a shot. She found Randy dead on the floor. George was telling Randy to wake up and play some more. No criminal negligence charges were ever pressed against the mother or her boyfriend. Instead, four-year-old George was put on a children's psychiatric ward, where he became the object of the staff's intense curiosity and analysis. He was soon receiving regular "play therapy."

Eighteen months later Joe Robinson and his new wife, Becky, were still trying to get George out of the psychiatric ward and into their own home. The Child Welfare Department, however, insisted that it should maintain custody of George, and the department based its opinion on the psychiatrists' opinions that George needed "continued residential treatment" because he was a "danger to himself and others." Psychiatry was, in other words, as willing to find murderous intent in a boy of four as it was willing to deny murderous intent in a coldblooded assassin like Dan White.

When the Robinsons began to contest the official opinions, the Child Welfare Department brought in an outside psychiatrist to offer a second opinion. He concluded that

George indeed needed "intensive therapy to help him work out his feelings about the shooting." This would require continued psychiatric hospitalization, since, in the words of the psychiatrist, "it would not be safe to turn my back on him for two minutes."

At this point I received a request from the Robinsons' attorney to look into the case. After meeting with young George and reviewing the opinions of the several psychiatrists, I concluded that the "experts" had gotten carried away. Common sense told me that at four years of age, George's shooting of his brother did not result from an intent to kill, but was purely an accident occurring during childish experimentation and play. He was no more "dangerous" than any other child.

It can be argued, of course, that the other psychiatrists were right and I was wrong. At the subsequent hearing, I urged the juvenile court judge to recognize that neither they nor I had any "special" tools to determine what young George was thinking at the time of the shooting. The judge should make up his own mind, I said, about whether George was the dangerous killer the other psychiatrists portrayed, or was instead the victim of adult negligence in leaving a loaded gun within reach of a young child. The judge sent George home with his father and the last I heard the child was doing fine, even without further "intensive therapy."

This case illustrates that psychiatric opinions affecting the lives of children are no more scientific than psychiatric opinions affecting the lives of adults. In cases of possible child neglect or abuse, indeed, psychiatrists' or psychologists' "examinations" and "tests" offer no greater insights or answers to crucial questions than the ordinary caseworker might provide.

Because psychiatric opinions are treated as though they were true medical findings, judges rarely question them. In the case of young George, he would have spent at least another year in an institution if his father's attorney hadn't called me to review the opinions of the other doctors. In most cases, no such rebuttal testimony is introduced, and a judge will accept psychiatrists' opinions as more or less definitive. Even when differing psychiatric opinions nullify each other, forcing a judge to resolve the issue alone, government agencies spend tax dollars for psychiatric input that is not special or "expert."

The older child in need of care and protection presents different problems. Whereas young children need adults to make choices for them, adolescents are capable of participating in decisionmaking. Just as with mental patients, teen-agers may not always make wise choices, but family members or child welfare caseworkers often do worse. *I recommend that the state no longer forcefully intervene in the lives of teen-agers considered "beyond parental control."*[28] Instead, voluntary shelters and community placements should be made available to them. Adolescents who believe they can support themselves should be allowed to do so, free from state interference. As sociologist Meda Chesney-Lind has said,

> There is a pressing need for runaway shelters, halfway houses and other community resources to deal with problems in a non-judicial context. Parents and children who are in conflict with society during adolescence should have resources available to them for their voluntary use.[29]

A number of communities have taken steps in this direction. Several states have prohibited the incarceration of status offenders, but none has gone so far as to completely remove truancy, running away, or incorrigibility from the jurisdiction of the juvenile court.[30] This step would be beneficial in two fundamental ways. First, it would enhance the rights of children, particularly girls. Second, it would open the way for more active experimentation with other alternatives. Addressing the juvenile court community, Judge David Bazelon put it well: "Because you act, no one else does."[31] We rely so heavily on state inter-ference in the lives of these teen-agers that we neglect other alternatives.

Punishing the Juvenile Offender

Unlike the child welfare services, the proposed juvenile justice system would be solely concerned with the admin-istration of justice. It would be in the business of the punishment and control of youthful offenders, just as the criminal justice system should be for adults. Once we have created a separate juvenile justice system focusing ex-clusively on the criminal activity of minors, we would not need to apologize for punishing young persons. As with adults, the state would focus its attention on the ad-ministration of fair penalties for young offenders and would not attempt coercive "rehabilitation."[32]

The first and most obvious benefit of a clear crime-and-punishment rationale is that minors charged with crimes would receive full constitutional protections in the courtroom. This idea is hardly new, and we have made sig-nificant strides in this respect. But to the extent that juvenile courts still hand down "findings" rather than "ver-dicts" and deny that they punish children, children still receive fewer due-process protections than adults.

The second benefit is that juvenile offenders would be protected from involuntary psychiatric treatments. They certainly need protection as much as adults. As law pro-fessor Sanford Fox says, the child would have a "right to punishment":

> A child's right to be punished imports remedies for the shortcomings and abuses in the justice system that are inherent in the treatment philosophy . . . punishment clearly implies limits, whereas a treat-ment does not . . . once it is acknowledged . . . that a child is being punished on account of what he has done, common sense, common decency, and the

like, step in and impose limits that are familiar and basic to every system of ethics.[33]

By "limits," Professor Fox refers to checks not only on what the state may do to an individual young offender but also on what state intervention may do in general.

> Unlike the treatment and rehabilitation goal, punishment counsels that the smallest possible number of children be thrust into the system, not the largest. Punishment cannot be mistaken as a technique for locating junior beneficiaries of a public trust, as a treatment-based juvenile justice system has been so misunderstood.[34]

Instead, we would more honestly recognize that juvenile justice, no less than adult justice, is worth pursuing on its own terms. It need not be considered as a tool of "help" for the young criminal. This rhetoric is just as hypocritical with children as it is with adults. We should punish young criminals, just as we should punish older criminals, because the social order requires it. Our present social order may not be all that we wish, but it will only get worse if we fail to punish lawbreakers. Punishment is necessary (to quote Professor Fox once more), "not to provide benefits or to identify needs, but rather because the law has been broken, and for reasons mostly relating to public security." Punishment, he adds, is "a coercive response having little to do with the welfare of the lawbreaker."[35]

This does not imply that a twelve-year-old bicycle thief should be locked up with sixteen-year-old murderers and rapists. *Just as we should classify crimes by adults into broad categories and give a fixed penalty for each, we should classify crimes by juveniles.* The penalty set in a particular case would be based on the crime committed, the age of the child, and the past record of proven criminal acts.[36]

Young offenders, like older offenders or mental patients, deserve the opportunity to accept or reject helping services. Voluntary services, however, should not result in mental evaluations that may influence the state's official response. We have an obligation to offer help because we as members of our society have had a hand in creating the social conditions that make delinquency more common in some neighborhoods than in others. And like adults, juvenile offenders will make better use of the help available when it is completely voluntary.

CHAPTER 12

CONCLUSIONS

I have tried to demonstrate that whenever psychiatry is given state power, no one is well served. It is simply too easy for psychiatric authority to become a vehicle of social policy more than a system of individual help. We do not need to use psychiatry in this way. We need instead a complete separation of state power and psychiatry. If this divorce were accomplished, the criminal justice system would do a better job of law enforcement, the courts would do a better job of deciding civil and criminal questions, and psychiatry would finally be free to offer honest and voluntary services to those who want help.

Until now we have mixed up these tasks, with unfortunate results. We have done so because we harbor two mistaken beliefs about psychiatry and social problems. First, we believe that if we act with enough good will, then involuntary psychiatric treatment can bring genuine help to unwilling recipients. I hope I have raised serious doubts about this belief.

Our second mistaken belief is one that I want to explore briefly before closing. It is commonly held that if we tamper with the minds and bodies of deviant persons, society will also be improved. We tell ourselves that if we rehabilitate enough criminals, we can reduce the rate of crime, and that if we promptly diagnose and treat enough mental patients, we can reduce the rate of mental disorder. But this approach has never reduced the incidence of either crime or mental disorder, and it never will. Help offered to individuals is one thing; help offered in the belief that we can thereby reduce the rate of crime or mental disorder is quite another and is doomed to failure. We pay a high price for our unrealistic expectations. The more we expect the remodeling of individuals to reduce the overall rates of mental disorder and crime, the more we neglect real solutions.

Divorcing psychiatry from all state authority might thus encourage us to develop genuine solutions to these problems. Without psychiatric pronouncements to disguise our ethical and social problems, we might be more willing to start the long and painful process of real social change.

Let us consider the problem of violence, as an example. Once we give up the idea that rehabilitating criminals will reduce volence, then perhaps we will seriously approach the problem from the more valid economic and political, rather than medical, perspective. Instead of trying to protect ourselves from violence by expecting psychiatrists to detect and treat dangerous persons, we might focus more attention on those dangerous *situations* that we could alter. Most murder victims in America, for example, are killed by people they know, not by criminals. The murderers are friends, lovers, or neighbors. I believe it is the ready availability of handguns that escalates family or neighborhood disputes into lethal violence. We are concerned about our appalling murder rate, yet we do nothing about the weapons that flood our society.

The medical community teaches that alcoholism is a disease, and spends millions of our tax dollars each year for research on its causes and cures. Yet this approach has been a failure. Moreover, it is likely to encourage problem drinkers to assume a passive and nonresponsible attitude toward their drinking. Patients, after all, are not ordinarily held responsible for their diseases. This "disease" model is good for doctors, but bad for society. It does not help alcoholics confront their addiction or help society confront its role in promoting alcoholic excess. This model, in fact, encourages society to ignore those policies that might

reduce the problem. Why not, for example, ban all adver-
tising of alcoholic beverages? Why not make a thirty-day
jail sentence *mandatory* for first-offense drunk drivers.
Second offenders would go to jail for one year and lose
their drivers' licenses for five years. Third offenders would
go to state prison for five years. The point is not to control
drinking with jail sentences, but to control *drunk driving*
with penalties that send a clear message to our people.
Many who drink and drive are not alcoholics and will control such behavior if the penalty is sufficient. We glamorize
alcohol at every turn, and should not be surprised when it
comes back to haunt us. Consider, for example, the fact
that half the deaths due to crime and accidents are alcohol
related.

As long as we cling to the hope that a better criminal
justice system will reduce violence, and that a better
mental health system will reduce mental disorder or
alcoholism, we will be less likely to initiate those social
and economic reforms that *could* reduce the problems.
We should, instead, be working on three independent
fronts, each with its own legitimacy, its own purposes
and methods.

First, we must design and implement social reforms
aimed at bringing more economic and political justice to
our people. These pose immensely difficult, long-term
problems, but such reforms are nonetheless the only way
to reduce the incidence of emotional breakdown and
criminal behavior.

Second, we must support and improve an honest criminal justice system aimed at controlling and punishing those
persons convicted of crimes. Its purpose would not be to
make society "better" or to "help" the criminal, but to
maintain the social order.

Third, we must establish a totally voluntary mental
health system, completely separate from any state power
and from the criminal justice system and the courts. It
would be aimed only at helping persons in emotional dis-
tress. While its helping purpose would be entirely legiti-

mate, it would not aim at improving society or reducing the overall incidence of mental disorder. Only social change will do that.

Each of these three goals is important. No one can be overlooked. Similarly, no one goal can take on the role of the other two. Needy persons deserve help, even though it will not change the social conditions causing most of the need. Criminals deserve, and society has a right to impose, fair punishment for lawbreaking, even though punishment will not change the social conditions that cause crime.

If we sincerely intend to confront the problems leading to mental disorder we must be prepared to make real social change. I believe that poverty is the most important single cause of major mental breakdown. More money in the pockets of more people, even if this means less money in the pockets of some of the people, would do more to reduce psychosis, violence, and suicide than a vast army of psychiatrists. This means reforms aimed at combating unemployment, racism, and corporate power. Members of any ideal society will, nonetheless, have their share of emotional troubles. But the *degree* to which such problems exist is, I believe, overwhelmingly determined by economic and political injustice.

Mental health professionals should not feel slighted by this analysis. If the mental health and criminal justice systems will never reduce the incidence of mental disorder and crime, this does not mean that professionals cannot help individuals. Psychiatrists can offer substantial help to troubled persons. When we free mental health professionals from all state power, they will finally be able to offer far more help than they do now.

It has been a terrible mistake to attack the problems of deviant behavior by arming psychiatry with state power, and there is no reason we cannot end this practice now. However tempting it is to continue our currently convenient relationship with psychiatry, we should gather the courage to disarm psychiatry and meet our social problems honestly.

NOTES

SELECTED BIBLIOGRAPHY

INDEX

NOTES

Introduction

1. I arrive at this total in the following way: California statistics indicate that each year seventy-five thousand persons are forcibly admitted to mental hospitals. These are formal, involuntary commitments. For each one, there are several more in which patients are pressured to "sign in" in order to avoid a formal commitment. A conservative estimate would therefore be 150,000 to 200,000 coercive admissions per year in California. Since California has one-tenth of the nation's people, we arrive at a national figure of 1.5 million to 2 million involuntary admissions per year in the United States.

2. This results from a finding of "incompetent to stand trial," the subject of chapter 5. A leading student of competency hearings, Henry Steadman, estimates that nine thousand persons are so labeled each year in the United States. See Henry Steadman, *Beating a Rap?: Defendants Found Incompetent to Stand Trial* (Chicago: University of Chicago Press, 1979), p. 4.

3. George Jackson, *Soledad Brother: The Prison Letters of George Jackson* (New York: Bantam Books, 1970).

4. Karl Menninger, *The Crime of Punishment* (New York: Viking Press, 1966).

Chapter 1. The Reign of Error

1. *San Francisco Chronicle*, August 2, 1975.

2. Alfred Freedman and Harold Kaplan, *Comprehensive Textbook of Psychiatry* (Baltimore: Williams and Wilkins, 1967), p. 504.

3. In the ordinary hospital or clinic setting, results of psychological testing are seldom challenged. In recent years, however, their increasing use in civil and criminal courts has led to several important reviews summarizing the literature. See Stephen J. Morse,

"Crazy Behavior, Morals, and Science: An Analysis of Mental Health Law," *Southern California Law Review* 51 (May 1978): 527; Jay Ziskin, *Coping with Psychiatric and Psychological Testimony*, 3rd ed. (Venice, Calif.: Law and Psychology Press, 1981). Even if psychological tests were reliable in a clinical context, this still would not alter the fact that "there are virtually no psychological tests that were designed for the purpose of measuring or assessing a legal issue" (Ziskin, p. 201).

4. Ziskin, pp. 216-224.

5. Ibid., pp. 225-242.

6. James Lawler, *I.Q., Heritability, and Racism* (New York: International Publishers, 1978). See also Stephen Jay Gould, *The Mismeasure of Man* (New York: W. W. Norton, 1981).

7. Ivan Illich, *Medical Nemesis: The Expropriation of Health* (New York: Random House, 1976).

8. Lee Coleman, "Problem Kids and Preventive Medicine: The Making of an Odd Couple," *American Journal of Orthopsychiatry* 48 (January 1978): 56.

9. Gould, pp. 222-233.

10. Alan Stone, *Mental Health and Law: A System in Transition*, Publication no. 76-176 (Washington, D.C.: U.S. Department of Health, Education, and Welfare, 1975), pp. 25-40.

11. Ellsworth Fersch, *Psychology and Psychiatry in Courts and Corrections* (New York: Wiley-Interscience, 1980), pp. 84-93.

12. Henry Steadman, "The Psychiatrist as a Conservative Agent of Social Control," *Social Problems* 20 (Fall 1972): 263.

13. John Monahan, "The Prevention of Violence," in John Monahan, ed., *Community Mental Health and the Criminal Justice System* (New York: Pergamon, 1975), p. 13.

14. People *v.* "George Chapman," Alameda County Superior Court, No. 69575-A.

15. Burke Smith, "The Polygraph," *Scientific American*, 216, no. 1 (January 1967): 25.

16. An example of how amobarbital (Amytal) interviews may be used to defend murderers was presented by Michael Sands, the defendant's attorney, in a paper entitled "The Mad Murderer in the Courtroom: Paul and Jack, a Case Study," at the American Psychiatric Association annual convention, New Orleans, May 11, 1981. Sands says, "Paul Miskimen was a hard-working, well-liked responsible citizen in Sacramento, California. In August 1979 he killed his wife, La Vaugn, for no apparent reason.

Psychiatric and psychological examination, including the use of sodium amytal and hypnosis, revealed that Paul had a separate distinct personality named Jack Kelly, and that Jack had forced Paul to commit the killing. In court Paul was found to be not guilty by reason of insanity." Here is the dialogue that allowed the doctors "almost accidentally" to discover "Jack Kelly, a distinct and separately identifiable personality living within the body of Paul Miskimen."

DOCTOR: Paul, why did you ask the clerk where you were?
DEFENDANT: I didn't know where I was.
DOCTOR: Were you confused?
DEFENDANT: I was confused.
DOCTOR: Did you know who you were?
DEFENDANT: Sure.
DOCTOR: Who were you?
DEFENDANT: Jack.
DOCTOR: Jack who?
DEFENDANT: Jack Kelly.

For more on narcoanalysis, see Carl Adatto, "Observations on Criminal Patients during Narcoanalysis," *Archives of Neurology and Psychiatry* 62 (1949): 82; Martin Gerson and Victor Victoroff, "Experimental Investigation into Validity of Confessions Obtained under Sodium Amytal Narcosis," *Journal of Clinical Psychopathology* 9 (1948): 359; W. F. Lorenz, "Criminal Confessions under Narcosis," *Wisconsin Medical Journal* 31 (1932): 245.

17. For an account in support of hypnosis as a fact finder, see Eugene Block, *Hypnosis: A New Tool in Crime Detection* (New York: David McKay, 1976).

18. The question of testimony from hypnotized witnesses has been discussed by the California Supreme Court in *People v. Donald Lee Shirley*, 31 Cal. 3d 18 (1982).

19. Bernauer Newton, "Procedures and Problems in Forensic Hypnosis" (Paper presented to the American Society for Clinical Hypnosis annual meeting, November 13, 1980), p. 4.

20. Bill Farr, "Bianchi under Hypnosis: Four Personalities Emerge," *Los Angeles Times,* December 26, 1979, p. 1.

21. "Was It Hypnosis or Hype?" *Time*, January 14, 1980, p. 50.

22. Too little data are available on how much we spend on courtroom evaluations by psychiatrists and psychologists. But William Farr, in "Jerry Hits Psychiatric Costs in Court Trials," *Los Angeles Times,* June 29, 1976, pt. 2, p. 1, writes, "One psychi-

atrist made $106,000 performing evaluations of accused crimi-
nals for the Los Angeles County Superior Court last year [1975].
Also $484,000 was paid in 1975 just to the 25 psychiatrists who
serve on the countywide panel that conducts psychiatric evaluations for Los Angeles County." Five years later the chairman of
the Psychiatric Panel Committee of Los Angeles County wrote,
"This year one doctor was paid approximately $81,000 during
the first six months of 1980" (personal correspondence).

23. American Psychiatric Association, *Diagnostic and Statistical
Manual of Mental Disorders*, 2d ed. (Washington, D.C.: American
Psychiatric Association, 1968), p. ix.

24. Ibid.

25. American Psychiatric Association, *Diagnostic and Statistical
Manual of Mental Disorders*, 3d ed. (Washington, D.C.: American
Psychiatric Association, 1980).

26. Robert Spitzer, et al., "Research Diagnostic Criteria," *Archives of
General Psychiatry* 35 (June 1978): 772.

27. For a summary of these developments, and a critique of the
third edition of the *Diagnostic and Statistical Manual*, see Jonas
Robitscher, *The Powers of Psychiatry* (Boston: Houghton Mifflin, 1980), chap. 11. Robitscher concludes, "Like a number of
other observers, I feel that the APA's new diagnostic system
does not represent an improvement, and that it does demonstrate publicly the inconsistencies of psychiatric thought and
increasingly unscientific and pragmatic nature of diagnostic
classification . . . the scheme does not rise to the scientific level
of the remainder of medicine, the studies used to support the
changes are often far from scientifically precise, and the fact
that the changes can be made at will and that social, political
and economic reasons are involved in the change all weaken psychiatry's claims to a scientific nomenclature" (p. 182). See also
Ziskin, pp. 130-158; Morse, pp. 543-554; and Daniel Goleman,
"Who's Mentally Ill?" *Psychology Today*, January 1978, p. 34.

28. *Diagnostic and Statistical Manual*, 3d ed., pp. 281-282 and 380.
When a homosexual expresses discontent with his sex life, the
manual tells us, he suffers from "Ego-dystonic homosexuality."
The desire to change must be "a persistent concern." See also
"A Symposium—Should Homosexuality Be in the APA Nomenclature?" *American Journal of Psychiatry* 130 (November
1973): 1207.

29. See Morse. See also Ziskin, chaps. 5-8. See also Bruce Ennis and
Thomas Litwack, "Psychiatry and the Presumption of Expertise," *California Law Review* 62 (May 1974): 693.

30. David Rosenhan, "On Being Sane in Insane Places," *Science* 179 (January 1973): 250. The most frequently cited critique of Rosenhan's experiment is Robert Spitzer, "On Pseudoscience in Science, Logic in Remission, and Psychiatric Diagnosis: A Critique of Rosenhan's 'On Being Sane in Insane Places,'" *Journal of Abnormal Psychology* 84 (1975): 442.

31. Morse, pp. 543 and 578.

Chapter 2. Hidden Agendas

1. Dr. Grigson's testimony in death penalty hearings is discussed in more detail in Jonas Robitscher, *The Powers of Psychiatry* (Boston: Houghton Mifflin, 1980), pp. 199–204. See also William Winslade, *The Insanity Plea: The Uses and Abuses of the Insanity Defense* (New York: Charles Scribner's, 1983), pp. 133–158.

2. *Texas Code of Criminal Procedure*, Supp. 1976–1977, Art. 37.071.

3. J. Bloom, "Doctor for the Prosecution," *American Lawyer*, November 1979, p. 26.

4. *Barefoot v. Estelle*, --U.S.--, 103 S.Ct.3383, 77 L. Ed. 2d 1090 (1983).

5. Ibid., p. 14.

6. Ibid., p. 16.

7. For more on psychiatry in death penalty hearings, see G. Dix, "The Death Penalty: 'Dangerousness,' Psychiatric Testimony, and Professional Ethics," *American Journal of Criminal Law* 5 (May 1977): 151, and G. Dix, "Participation by Mental Health Professionals in Capital Murder Sentencing," *International Journal of Law and Psychiatry* 1 (1978): 283.

8. Martin Lipp, *The Bitter Pill: Doctors, Patients, and Failed Expectations* (New York: Harper and Row, 1980).

9. Ibid., p. 101.

10. Ibid.

11. Ibid., p. 99.

12. Ibid.

13. Robitscher, p. 401.

14. Lipp, p. 10.

Chapter 3. The Insanity Defense

1. Carolyn Anspacher, *The Trial of Dr. De Kaplany* (New York: Frederick Fell, 1965). All quotations and data on this trial are drawn from this book.

2. Ibid., p. 22.
3. Ibid., p. 17.
4. Ibid., p. 115.
5. Ibid., p. 125.
6. Ibid., p. 80.
7. Ibid., p. 81.
8. Ibid., p. 96.
9. Ibid., p. 101.
10. Ibid., p. 98.
11. California State Senate, and California State Assembly, Joint Committee on Revision of the Penal Code, *Hearings on the Role of Psychiatry in Determining Criminal Responsibility*, April 11 and April 12, 1979, pp. 24-25.
12. T. George Harris, "Psychiatrist Bernard L. Diamond Tells of the Bizarre Paranoia He Found in Sirhan B. Sirhan: A Conversation with T. George Harris," *Psychology Today*, September 1969, p. 48.
13. Ibid., p. 50.
14. Ibid.
15. William Winslade, *The Insanity Plea: The Uses and Abuses of the Insanity Defense* (New York: Charles Scribner's, 1983), p. 3.
16. For an overview of the different approaches to defining legal insanity, see Alexander Brooks, *Law, Psychiatry, and the Mental Health System* (Boston: Little, Brown, 1974), pp. 111-319.
17. For a description of this trial, by a leading advocate of psychiatric testimony, see Bernard Diamond, "Isaac Ray and the Trial of Daniel M'Naughten," *American Journal of Psychiatry* (February 1956): 651.
18. Anthony Platt and Bernard Diamond, "Origins of the 'Right and Wrong' Test of Criminal Responsibility and Its Subsequent Development in the United States: An Historical Survey," *California Law Review* 54 (1966): 1227.
19. Isaac Ray, *A Treatise on the Medical Jurisprudence of Insanity* (Boston: Little, Brown, 1838).
20. Philip Roche, *The Criminal Mind* (New York: Grove Press, 1958), pp. 176-177.
21. *Durham v. United States* 214 F.2d 862 (D.C. Cir. 1954).
22. Brooks, p. 177.
23. American Law Institute, *Model Penal Code* (1962).
24. *United States v. Brawner* 471 F.2d 979 (D.C. Cir. 1972).
25. Court-martial of "Tony," U.S. Air Force File # 8019D6-508.

26. Winslade, p. 200.
27. See Nigel Walker, *Crime and Insanity in England* (Edinburgh: Edinburgh University Press, 1968). See also Platt and Diamond.
28. For data on length of incarceration, see Henry Steadman, "Insanity Acquittals in New York State, 1965-1978," *American Journal of Psychiatry* 137 (March 1980): 321. Also Anne Singer, "Insanity Acquittals in the Seventies: Observations and Empirical Analysis of One Jurisdiction," *Mental Disability Law Reporter* 2 (1978): 406.
29. Steadman, p. 325.
30. Singer. p. 407.
31. Steadman, p. 322.
32. *Chicago Tribune*, April 18, 1978.
33. Ibid.
34. For a discussion of Edmund Kemper, by a leading forensic psychiatrist, see Donald Lunde, *Murder and Madness* (Stanford, Calif.: The Portable Stanford, 1975), pp. 53-55.
35. Lee Coleman, "Perspectives on the Medical Research of Violence," *American Journal of Orthopsychiatry* 44 (October 1974): 675. See also Alan Scheflin and Edward Opton, *The Mind Manipulators* (New York: Paddington Press, 1978), pp. 266-324, for a critical assessment of psychosurgical procedures sometimes advocated for alleged "violence-producing epilepsy." See also Antonio V. Delgado-Escueta, et al., "Special Report: The Nature of Aggression during Epileptic Seizures," *New England Journal of Medicine* 305 (September 17, 1981): 711.
36. Torsney's case has now been extensively covered. See Susan Sheehan, "The Patient: Part I—Creedmoor Psychiatric Center," *The New Yorker*, May 25, 1979, p. 75. See also Winslade, pp. 133-158.
37. *National Enquirer*, December 9, 1977.
38. *In re Moye* 22 Cal. 3d 457 (1978).
39. For a summary of the evidence, see Saleem Shah, "Dangerousness and Civil Commitment of the Mentally Ill: Some Public Policy Considerations," *American Journal of Psychiatry* 132 (May 1975): 501.
40. American Psychiatric Association Insanity Defense Work Group, *Statement on the Insanity Defense* (Washington, D.C.: American Psychiatric Association, 1982).
41. Ibid., p. 11.
42. Ibid., p. 16.

Chapter 4. Diminished Capacity

1. For a more detailed account of the political events leading to the assassinations, see Warren Hinckle, "Dan White's San Francisco," *Inquiry*, October 29, 1979, p. 8.

2. Some observers of the White trial, such as Hinckle, place the entire blame for the outcome on what they see as an inept and even corrupt team of prosecutors. It is Hinckle's contention that because the San Francisco law enforcement community did not want its antigay attitudes exposed at the trial, prosecutors failed to develop the political motivations behind White's killings. Whether or not these allegations are true, it was the psychiatric testimony and the tortured definitions of "diminished capacity" that overwhelmed the jury's common sense.

3. The quotations cited are from the transcript of the trial, graciously próvided to me by Thomas Norman, assistant district attorney of San Francisco County.

4. For a discussion of the development of the case law of diminished capacity, see Stephen Morse, "Diminished Capacity: A Moral and Legal Conundrum," *International Journal of Law and Psychiatry* 2 (1979): 271.

5. Bernard Diamond, "Criminal Responsibility of the Mentally Ill," *Stanford Law Review* 14 (1961): 59.

6. Ibid., p. 61.

7. Ibid., p. 62.

8. The facts of the *Wells* case, as well as the role of psychiatric testimony during the appeal and the reasoning of the court, may be found in the California Supreme Court decision. See *People v. Wells* 33 Cal. 2d 330 (1949).

9. Section 4500 of the *California Penal Code* at that time stated, "Every person undergoing a life sentence in a State Prison of this state, who with malice aforethought commits an assault on the person of another with a deadly weapon or instrument, or by any means of force likely to produce great bodily injury, is punishable by death." This law was undoubtedly a response to the fear of prison officials that without the threat of death, a "lifer" could assault guards or other prisoners and have "nothing to lose." Because California courts had ruled in *People v. McNabb* (3 Cal. 2d 441 [1935]) and *People v. Williams* (27 Cal. 2d 216 [1945]) that even a prisoner with a sentence like six months to life had been given a "life sentence," this law meant that even persons with no previous history of violence could be put to death.

10. 338 U.S. 836 (1949), cert. denied.

11. *People v. Gorshen* 51 Cal. 2d 716 (1959).

12. Diamond, p. 75, n. 51.

13. Ibid., pp. 76-77.

14. Diamond admitted as much in his 1961 *Stanford Law Review* article. He wrote, "By all conventional rules of law, a conviction of first degree murder was inevitable." See Diamond, p. 77.

15. Ibid., pp. 77-78.

16. Ibid., p. 78.

17. *People v. Gorshen,* p. 722.

18. Ibid., p. 723.

19. George Olhausen, *Amicus Brief,* filed November 26, 1958, in *People v. Gorshen,* on behalf of the eighteen prominent psychiatrists.

20. Ibid., p. 7.

21. Diamond, p. 82.

22. As of 1982, ten states had some form of diminished capacity law, according to an informal survey conducted by the California legislature's Joint Committee on Revision of the Penal Code; the results of the survey were personally communicated to me by counsel to the committee, Edward Cohen. Many more states, however, permit such testimony, even though no special laws relating to diminished capacity are on the books. For a review of these developments, see Robert Park Bryant and Corbin Brooke Hume, "Diminished Capacity—Recent Decisions and an Analytic Approach," *Vanderbilt Law Review* 30 (1977): 213. While this article provides a good review of diminished capacity case law, it also—unwisely, I believe—promotes the role of psychiatry in determinations of criminal responsibility. See also Peter Arenella, "The Diminished Capacity and Diminished Responsibility Defenses: Two Children of a Doomed Marriage," *Columbia Law Review* 77 (October 1977): 827.

23. Phillip E. Johnson, "The Supreme Court of California, 1975-1976: Foreword—The Accidental Decision and How It Happens," *California Law Review* 65 (1977): 242.

24. Arenella, p. 844.

25. This language, which law professor Phillip Johnson has aptly described as "impenetrable," is from the opinion of California Supreme Court Justice Roger Traynor in *People v. Conley* 64 Cal. 2d 310 (1966).

26. Once again, it was the California Supreme Court, not the California legislature, that was responsible for this burdensome and vague language. See *People v. Wolff* 61 Cal. 2d (1964) at 818–823.

27. Dino Fulgoni, "Medieval Systematics in the Modern Law of Crime," *Prosecutor's Brief, Journal of the California District Attorneys Association* 3 (January–February 1980): 10.

28. Jim Wood, *The Rape of Inez Garcia* (New York: Putnam's, 1976), pp. 148–149.

Chapter 5. Incompetent to Stand Trial

1. For a discussion of the hypocritical roots of competency hearings, see Abraham Halpern, "Use and Misuse of Psychiatry in Competency Examinations of Criminal Defendants," *Psychiatric Annals* 5.4 (April 1975): 8. Halpern discusses the fact that the *parens patriae* (the state as parent) doctrine was a self-serving policy from the beginning, in both Roman and medieval English law. Halpern recommends that competence-for-trial hearings be abolished, but leaves the door open for civil commitment to be used in its place. This is a solution I find unacceptable.

2. This fact is by now recognized by virtually all students of the subject. For moving accounts of such lawlessness and how it can affect the individuals caught in it, see Bruce Ennis, *Prisoners of Psychiatry* (New York: Avon Books, 1972). See also Thomas Szasz, *Psychiatric Justice* (Westport, Conn.: Greenwood Press, 1965).

3. Halpern, p. 9.

4. For clear evidence of this, see Henry Steadman, *Beating a Rap?: Defendants Found Incompetent to Stand Trial* (Chicago: University of Chicago Press, 1979).

5. Ralph Slovenko, *Psychiatry and Law* (Boston: Little, Brown, 1973), p. 96.

6. Steadman, generally.

7. Ibid., p. 52.

8. Ibid., p. 34.

9. Group for the Advancement of Psychiatry, *Misuse of Psychiatry in the Criminal Courts: Competency to Stand Trial*, Vol. 8, Report no. 89 (New York: Group for the Advancement of Psychiatry, 1974), p. 884.

10. For an interesting account of the psychiatric debacle in the Hearst trial, see Shana Alexander, *Anyone's Daughter* (New York: Viking Press, 1979).
11. See Ennis for examples of this in actual courtroom testimony. A landmark study revealing this fact is Louis McGarry, "Demonstration and Research in Competency for Trial and Mental Illness: Review and Preview," *Boston University Law Review* 49 (1969): 46.
12. Steadman, p. 15. Jonas Robitscher in *The Powers of Psychiatry* (Boston: Houghton Mifflin, 1980) gives an example (p. 26) of how these practices can degenerate into a nightmare of lawlessness. Four soldiers had been accused of murder. Three were convicted and the fourth was found incompetent to stand trial. Then, all four were found to have been improperly tried. As a result, Robitscher tells us, "three were set free, but the fourth, who had been declared incompetent to stand trial, was held in a hospital for the criminally insane because he did not have the capacity to participate in the proceeding to have his indictment dismissed."
13. McGarry, p. 50.
14. Ibid., pp. 51–52.
15. Ibid., p. 52.
16. Ibid., p. 56.
17. Editors, "Comment: Commitment to Farview: Incompetency to Stand Trial," *University of Pennsylvania Law Review* 117 (1969): 1164.
18. S. L. Stebel, *The Shoe Leather Treatment* (Los Angeles: J. P. Tarcher/St. Martin's Press, 1980).
19. Ibid., p. 92.
20. *In re Thomas Spychala*, Crim. No. 21338, California Supreme Court, January 30, 1980. Petition denied March 18, 1980.
21. *Jackson v. Indiana* 406 U.S. 715 (1972).
22. Ibid.
23. Ibid.
24. See Halpern for some examples of how the states have responded to the *Jackson* decision.
25. See Marjory Parker, "California's New Scheme for the Commitment of Individuals Found Incompetent to Stand Trial," *Pacific Law Journal* 6 (July 1975): 484, for a sympathetic account of these developments in California.

26. *In re Davis* 8 Cal. 3d 798 (1973).
27. All quotations from R. T.'s case are from his medical records at Napa State Hospital, Imola, California.
28. *State v. Rodriguez*, Circuit Court, 1st District of Hawaii, 53619.

Chapter 6. A Matter of Consent

1. See Richard Hunter and Ida MacAlpine, *Three Hundred Years of Psychiatry: 1535-1860* (London: Oxford University Press, 1963), p. 662.
2. Charles Goshen, ed., *Documentary History of Psychiatry* (New York: Philosophical Library, 1967), pp. 278 and 274.
3. Ibid., p. 280.
4. For a closer look at Freeman's work, see Walter Freeman, James Watts, and Thelma Hunt, *Psychosurgery: Intelligence, Emotion, and Social Behavior following Prefrontal Lobotomy for Mental Disorders* (Springfield, Ill.: Charles C Thomas, 1942).
5. See David Shutts, *Lobotomy: Resort to the Knife* (New York: Van Nostrand Reinhold, 1982).
6. John Pfeiffer, "Medicine's Good News for Sick Minds." This article was sent to me with the date and source not included. I have been unable to track it down, but the article was clearly written for a lay audience. From the jacket of his book *The Human Brain* (New York: Harper, 1955), we learn that Pfeiffer wrote for such prestigious magazines as *Scientific American*, *Harper's*, and *New York Times Magazine*. He was clearly a leading science writer. Hence, his unstinting praise for lobotomy was a reflection of what many of our best people, both professional and lay, were thinking and writing.
7. See note 4 for the first edition. For the second edition, see Walter Freeman, James Watts, and Mary Frances Robinson, *Psychosurgery: In the Treatment of Mental Disorders and Intractable Pain* (Springfield, Ill.: Charles C Thomas, 1950).
8. Quoted in Charles Steir, ed., *Blue Jolts: True Stories from the Cuckoo's Nest* (Washington, D.C.: New Republic Books, 1978), p. 130.
9. See Max Rinkel and Harold Himwich, eds., *Insulin Treatment in Psychiatry* (New York: Philosophical Library, 1959). See also Manfred Sakel, *Schizophrenia* (New York: Philosophical Library,

1958). See also Manfred Sakel, "The Classical Sakel Shock Treatment: A Reappraisal," in A. Sackler, et al., *The Great Physiodynamic Therapies in Psychiatry: An Historical Reappraisal* (New York: Hoeber-Harper, 1956), pp. 13–75. I know of no better way to understand the horror experienced by many institutionalized mental patients than a careful reading of books like these, which are filled with the most fantastic theories of and remedies for mental disorder.

10. Sackler, et al., p. 20.

11. For Meduna's own account, see Laszlo Meduna, "The Convulsive Treatment: A Reappraisal," in Sackler, et al., p. 76. Listen to how Meduna rationalized his new method of shock treatment (p. 77). "I observed the extreme hyperplasia of the glia system in epileptic brains in contrast with the apparent torpor of the glia system in schizophrenic brains. To explain the difference in epilepsy and the behavior of these cells in schizophrenia, I developed the hypothesis that the noxa causing epilepsy has a stimulating effect upon the growth of the glia cells, while the noxa producing schizophrenia has an opposite, a paralyzing, effect on the glia system. Thus, fairly early, I developed an idea of some sort of antagonism between the behavior of the glia system in epilepsy and the behavior of this system in schizophrenia. Later, in about 1930, I became acquainted with Dr. Julius Nyiro, who told me that, in 1929, he had been interested in epilepsy and in its combination with schizophrenia and that he had found that schizophrenic processes have a benign effect upon the epileptic process . . . On the basis of his observations, Nyiro had assumed that the schizophrenic process must have a curative effect on the epilepsy and had begun his investigations on this probability by *transfusing schizophrenic blood into epileptic patients* . . . Nyiro did not even think of treating, conversely, schizophrenic patients by transfusing into them epileptic blood or by provoking in them epileptic attacks . . . I had only to find a convulsant drug which would produce epileptic attacks" (emphasis added).

12. For Cerletti's own account, see Ugo Cerletti, "Electroshock Therapy," in Sackler, et al., p. 91. For an invaluable resource on the history of electroshock treatment, see Leonard Frank, ed., *The History of Shock Treatment* (1978). This book is available directly from the editor, 2300 Webster St., San Francisco, Calif. 94115.

13. See American Psychiatric Association Task Force, *Electroconvulsive Therapy*, Report no. 14 (Washington, D.C.: American Psychiatric Association, 1978). Peter Breggin in *Electroshock:*

Its Brain-Disabling Effects (New York: Springer, 1979) agrees with this estimate. He agrees with little else in the American Psychiatric Association report. Breggin's account is the best one available, and is highly readable.

14. *Time*, November 19, 1976, p. 76.

15. For a summary of the evidence showing brain damage, see Breggin, pp. 74–101. See also John Friedberg, "Shock Treatment, Brain Damage, and Memory Loss: A Neurological Perspective," *American Journal of Psychiatry* 134 (September 1977): 1010.

16. See Breggin, pp. 114–122. He writes, "One reason the increased current is required in modern ECT is the use of barbiturates, which raise the seizure threshold." As a source for this important point, Breggin calls on a leading advocate of ECT, Lothar Kalinowsky. See Lothar Kalinowsky, "The Convulsive Therapies," in Alfred Freedman, Harold Kaplan, and Benjamin Sadock, eds., *Comprehensive Textbook of Psychiatry*, 2d ed. (Baltimore: Williams and Wilkins, 1975), p. 1971.

17. Sidney Sament, Letter to the Editor, *Clinical Psychiatry News*, March 1983, p. 4.

18. Even proponents of shock treatment admit it causes severe memory impairment in the weeks following the treatment. They claim, however, that this completely disappears in a month or two. For an account indicating that this is not so, see Marilyn Rice, "The Rice Papers," in Leonard Frank, ed., pp. 92–97. Berton Roueche has written an account of Rice's experiences: "As Empty as Eve," *The New Yorker*, September 9, 1974, p. 84.

19. The evidence that shock treatment can cause permanent intellectual impairment nonetheless comes not only from critics like Breggin or Friedberg but also from literature generally supportive of shock treatment. See, for example, American Psychiatric Association Task Force, *Report*, p. 58, where one reads that "impairment in learning new material . . . is cumulative with successive treatments."

20. Peter Breggin, "Coercion of Voluntary Patients in an Open Hospital," *Archives of General Psychiatry* 10 (February 1964): 173.

21. Eloise Dungan, in the *San Francisco Examiner*, November 12, 1972, quotes Leonard Cammer, a major advocate of shock treatment, as follows: "A depressed man or woman is like a car that can't turn the motor over with a weak battery. It needs a recharge." See Leonard Frank, ed., pp. 89–90, for more from this article.

22. This was the explanation given before a committee of the Hawaii state legislature by a psychiatrist testifying against legislation to regulate consent procedures for shock treatment. Hawaii, House of Representatives, Health Committee, Testimony on House Bill 1973 and Senate Bill 1710, February 13, 1978.

23. For an excellent account of these activities, see Alan Scheflin and Edward Opton, *The Mind Manipulators* (New York: Paddington Press, 1978), pp. 106-242. See also John Marks, *The Search for the Manchurian Candidate: The CIA and Mind Control* (New York: New York Times Books, 1979). Another book dealing with this subject, Walter Bowart's *Operation Mind Control* (New York: Dell, 1978), perpetuates the myth that the government was indeed able to create robots and zombies.

24. Howard Kahn and Martin Porter, "The Secret Army Drug Experiments: What Did Warren Burger Know?" *Rolling Stone*, April 21, 1977, p. 46. See also Scheflin and Opton, pp. 170-176.

25. Paul Hoch, "Experimentally Produced Psychoses," *American Journal of Psychiatry* 107 (February 1951): 607.

26. Nolan D. C. Lewis and Margaret O. Strahl, eds., *The Complete Psychiatrist: The Achievements of Paul H. Hoch, M.D.* (Albany: State University of New York Press, 1968).

27. D. Ewen Cameron, J. G. Lohrenz, and K. A. Handcock, "The Depatterning Treatment of Schizophrenia," *Comprehensive Psychiatry* 3 (April 1962): 65.

28. *DeClassified Documents News* 2.2 (1977): 1. This is available from Carrolton Press, Inc., Arlington, Virginia.

29. Two psychiatrists who did not miss the deeper lessons of the "mind control" exposé of 1975 are Thomas Szasz and Peter Breggin. See Thomas Szasz, "Patriotic Poisoners," *The Humanist* (November-December 1976): 5, and Peter Breggin, "Psychiatry and the CIA Connection," *Libertarian Review* (September 1979): 32.

Chapter 7. Psychiatry's New Drugs

1. For typical examples of current enthusiasm for biochemical explanations and treatments of mental disorders, from two leading psychiatrists, see Solomon Snyder, *Madness and the Brain* (New York: McGraw-Hill, 1974), and Ronald Fieve, *Moodswing: The Third Revolution in Psychiatry* (New York: William Morrow, 1975). For a critical review of this phenomenon, see Peter Sterling, "Psychiatry's Drug Addiction," *The New Republic*,

December 8, 1979, p. 14. A critique for professionals, but still highly readable, is Peter Breggin's *Psychiatric Drugs: Hazards to the Brain* (New York: Springer, 1983).

2. See, for example, Richard F. Mollica, "From Asylum to Community: The Threatened Disintegration of Public Psychiatry," *New England Journal of Medicine* 308 (February 17, 1983): 368.

3. While psychiatry likes to describe any drug-induced change in the patient as "improvement" or even "cure," other interpretations are worth considering. Psychiatrist Peter Breggin has written, "From 1954 through 1958 I . . . personally witnessed the 'miracle' wrought by the introduction of the major tranquilizers into the state mental hospitals . . . There can be no doubt about the effect of the medications. Prior to their introduction, electroshock treatment and insulin coma therapy were the mainstays of patient control. When an individual was difficult to manage within the confines of these foul-smelling, dilapidated, overcrowded concentration camps, he was involuntarily subjected to a brutal series of shocks or comas, often rendering him more tractable and more willing to hide his craziness or his rebellion. Nonetheless, the wards remained very unruly, and for the hospital staff they were often dangerous. But with the advent of the major tranquilizers a dramatic change took place. Instead of the traditional disorderly madhouse filled with upset, outraged inmates, we now had a storehouse filled with apathetic, robot-like non-persons. This was my personal introduction to the miracle of modern psychiatry." See Peter Breggin, "Brain-Disabling Therapies," in Elliot Valenstein, ed., *The Psychosurgery Debate: Scientific, Legal, and Ethical Perspectives* (San Francisco: W. H. Freeman, 1980), p. 476.

4. Many people have forgotten, or are too young to remember, the widespread public feeling in the 1950s that too much money was being spent on mental asylums. As the jacket cover of a popular book of the day proclaimed, "Every other hospital bed in the United States is occupied by a mental case. Mental illness costs this country two and a half billion dollars a year." See Mike Gorman, *Every Other Bed* (Cleveland, Oh.: World, 1956).

5. Andrew Scull in *Decarceration* (Englewood Cliffs, N.J.: Prentice-Hall, 1977) discusses the economic roots of deinstitutionalization of mental patients. See also Franklin Chu and Sharland Trotter, *The Madness Establishment* (New York: Grossman, 1974).

6. Personal conversation with Joseph O'Connor, November 21, 1980.

7. Sterling, p. 17.

8. Milton Silverman and Philip R. Lee, *Pills, Politics, and Profits* (Berkeley: University of California Press, 1974), pp. 27-31. Particularly informative is table 2 on page 328, which compares the profits of U.S. drug manufacturers and those of other U.S. manufacturers. During each year that the table covers (1960-1972), drug company profits (in percentages) were nearly twice those of other companies. These figures are for all types of drugs, not just psychiatric drugs. For a useful account of the "minor tranquilizer" market, see Richard Hughes and Robert Brewin, *The Tranquilizing of America* (New York: Harcourt Brace Jovanovich, 1979).

9. For a more detailed description of these goings-on, see June Noble and William Noble, *The Psychiatric Fix: Psychiatry's Alarming Power over Our Lives* (New York: Delacorte, 1981), pp. 245-254.

10. Ingrid Waldron, "Increased Prescribing of Valium, Librium, and Other Drugs—An Example of the Influence of Economic and Social Factors on the Practice of Medicine," *International Journal of Health Services* 7 (1977): 37.

11. Mitchell Balter and Mary Lou Bauer, "Patterns of Prescribing and Use of Hypnotic Drugs in the United States," in A. D. Clift, ed., *Sleep Disturbance and Hypnotic Drug Dependence* (Amsterdam: Excerpta Medica, 1975). Balter and Bauer write, "As with other classes of psychotropic drugs, general practitioners and internists are the chief prescribers of hypnotics" (p. 276). The situation is no different with the tranquilizers. See also J. Maurice Rogers, "Drug Abuse—Just What the Doctor Ordered," *Psychology Today*, September 1971, p. 16.

12. For a brief but excellent summary of this general problem, see Henry L. Lennard, Leon J. Epstein, Arnold Bernstein, and Donald C. Ransom, *Mystification and Drug Misuse* (New York: Perennial Library, 1971).

13. Scull, p. 79.

14. Sterling, p. 16.

15. See, for example, the summary of studies in John Davis, "Overview: Maintenance Therapy in Psychiatry: I. Schizophrenia," *American Journal of Psychiatry* 132 (December 1975): 1237. This article is seen by many in psychiatry as the definitive summary of the evidence that "chronic schizophrenics" must take antipsychotic drugs if they hope to avoid relapse. Yet of the twenty-four "controlled" studies cited, Davis admits that "in

many of these major studies chronic schizophrenic inpatients were used." This is a crucial admission, for what nurses and doctors on a psychiatric ward describe as "relapse" may simply mean that the patient is more difficult to manage. Patients who are not on these drugs are indeed more likely to be troublesome inmates on locked wards than are drugged patients. Studies of such persons *in the community* would be more useful, and Davis says that "there are also adequate data on schizophrenic outpatients," but does not tell us which (or how many) of the twenty-four studies were done on outpatients. Every example that Davis specifically describes, moreover, involved hospitalized patients. Davis also bluntly admits that "there have been no long-term studies on maintenance medication." Since Davis does not discuss any outpatient studies, only reassuring us that the studies exist, we cannot answer the crucial question of the studies—whether patients relapse because of lack of medication or because of other factors. For a comprehensive and critical review of the literature supporting maintenance medication, see L. L. Tobias and M. L. MacDonald, "Withdrawal of Maintenance Drugs with Long-Term Hospitalized Patients: A Critical Review," *Psychological Bulletin* 81 (1974): 107–125.

Ironically, the next issue of the *American Journal of Psychiatry* after that presenting Davis's paper contains another paper discussing the sloppy nature of those outpatient studies that do exist. George Gardos and Jonathan Cole, in "Maintenance Antipsychotic Therapy: Is the Cure Worse Than the Disease?" *American Journal of Psychiatry* (January 1976): 32, point out that many "relapses" brought on by stopping "antipsychotic" medication are in fact the result of the unmasking of brain damage induced by the medications.

16. The counterproductive impact of long-term medication has been studied by Maurice Rappaport, H. Kenneth Hopkins, Karyl Hall, Teodoro Belleza, and Julian Silverman in "Schizophrenics for Whom Phenothiazines May Be Contraindicated or Unnecessary," *International Pharmacopsychiatry* 13 (1978): 100. Patients given placebo (inert substance) were found to do better *after discharge* than those kept on chlorpromazine (Thorazine). *In the hospital*, however, the patients kept on chlorpromazine did "better" than the placebo group. This strongly suggests that what doctors and nurses consider "improvement" in a mental hospital is compliance rather than real capacity.

17. Wade Hudson, personal testimony. See U.S. Congress, Senate, Committee on the Judiciary, Subcommittee to Investigate Ju-

venile Delinquency, *Drugs in Institutions*, vol. 3, 94th Cong., 1st sess., 1975, p. 31.
18. Personal affidavit.
19. For a comprehensive review of these side effects, see Richard Shader and Alberto DiMascio, *Psychotropic Drug Side Effects* (Baltimore: Williams and Wilkins, 1970). For a discussion of the question of whether these drugs are truly "antipsychotic," see Breggin, *Psychiatric Drugs*, pp. 56-59.
20. David Raskin, "Akathisia: A Side Effect to Be Remembered," *American Journal of Psychiatry* 129 (September 1972): 121.
21. For a good summary of this problem, see Dr. Caligari (pen name of psychiatrist David Richman), "Psychiatric Drug Deaths," *On the Edge: Newsletter of the Bay Area Committee for Alternatives to Psychiatry* 2 (June 1981): 3. See also Allen Markman, "Death by Psychiatry: A Preliminary Review of Eight Deaths in the New York State Psychiatric System," *Phoenix Rising* 3 (Spring 1983): 5.
22. Frederick Zugibe, "Sudden Death Related to the Use of Psychotropic Drugs," in Cyril H. Wecht, ed., *Legal Medicine, 1980* (Philadelphia: W. B. Saunders, 1980), p. 25. See also Pranay Gupte, "Tranquilizers Held an Agent in Deaths of Mental Patients," *New York Times*, July 17, 1978, p. 1.
23. Gupte, p. 1.
24. Personal communication, August 6, 1982.
25. See Theodore Van Putten, "Why Do Schizophrenic Patients Refuse to Take Their Drugs?" *Archives of General Psychiatry* 31 (July 1974): 67. See also David E. Raskin, "Akathisia: A Side Effect to Be Remembered," *American Journal of Psychiatry* 129 (September 1972): 121.
26. Much credit goes to George Crane, director of research at Spring Grove State Hospital, Baltimore, for insisting that psychiatrists pay more attention to tardive dyskinesia. In "Clinical Psychopharmacology in Its Twentieth Year," *Science* 181 (July 13, 1973): 124, he wrote, "The psychiatric community has become more and more dependent on the use of neuroleptic agents. One of the consequences of this reliance on psychopharmacology has been the tendency to minimize the potential danger of long-term exposure to powerful chemical agents. Thus, permanent neurological disorders have become very common among patients treated with neuroleptics, but little effort has been made to come to grips with this problem." For an illustration of psychiatry's belated attempt to "come to grips" with the problem—by

268   THE REIGN OF ERROR

developing yet more drugs to "counteract" tardive dyskinesia—see American Psychiatric Association Task Force, "Tardive Dyskinesia: Summary of a Task Force Report of the American Psychiatric Association," *American Journal of Psychiatry* 137 (October 1980): 1163. The report argues that "an alarmist view is unwarranted."

27. Gardos and Cole, p. 35.
28. I chose this particular advertisement out of the thousands that have appeared because it is over twenty years old. See *Mental Hospitals* (May 1962): 263. In the two decades since, nothing has changed.
29. Daniel Chandler and Andrea Sallychild, *The Use and Misuse of Psychiatric Drugs in California's Mental Health Programs*, 31 (Sacramento: Assembly Office of Research, June 1977).
30. Ibid., p. 8.
31. Office of Planning and Program Analysis, California Department of Health, *Task Force Investigation of State Hospital Resident Deaths (1973-76)* (Sacramento, California Department of Health, June 15, 1978), p. 5.
32. Gupte, p. 1.
33. *Davis v. Hubbard* 506 F.Supp. 915 (N.D. Ohio, W.D. 1980). For a critical analysis of *Davis v. Hubbard*, see *Hamline Law Review* 4 (June 1981): 597.
34. *Rennie v. Klein* 462 F.Supp. 1131 (D. N.J. 1978).
35. *Rogers v. Okin* 478 F.Supp. 1342 (D. Mass. 1979). As of this writing, this case is still not settled. For a discussion of the case, see Breggin, *Psychiatric Drugs*, pp. 227-241.
36. John Latz and Gaye Jenkins, "Lithium: Miracle Drug or Emotional Straitjacket?" *State and Mind* (Spring 1978): 25.
37. Frank Ayd, "The Depot Fluphenazines: A Reappraisal after 10 Years' Clinical Experience," *American Journal of Psychiatry* 132 (May 1975): 491.
38. H. Lehmann, "The Philosophy of Long Acting Medication in Psychiatry," *Diseases of the Nervous System* 31 Supp. (September 1970): 7.
39. Jonas Robitscher, *The Powers of Psychiatry* (Boston: Houghton Mifflin, 1980), p. 359.
40. Fieve, p. 238.
41. For a review of lithium's toxic effects, from proponents of the drug, see Barry Reisberg and Samuel Gershon, "Side Effects Associated with Lithium Therapy," *Archives of General Psy-*

chiatry 36 (July 20, 1979): 879. For a review by two critics of lithium use, see Breggin, *Psychiatric Drugs,* pp. 185–224; and Dr. Caligari, "From Guinea Pig to Guinea Pig," *Madness Network News* 3 (December 1975): 11. The most ominous of lithium's side effects is permanent kidney damage after longterm use, the incidence of which is still in question. See Frederick Jenner, "Lithium and the Question of Kidney Damage," *Archives of General Psychiatry* 36 (July 20, 1979): 888.

42. While I have been focusing in this chapter mainly on schizophrenia and the major tranquilizers, or so-called antipsychotics, the overblown claims regarding biochemical etiology are similar in the case of the "affective" or mood disorders. See Boo Chiong, "The Evidence against the Catecholamine Hypothesis," *Psychiatric Opinion* (September 1979): 10.

43. Fieve, p. 225.

44. Frederick Goodwin, "Introduction to the Lithium Ion," *Archives of General Psychiatry* 36 (July 20, 1979): 834.

45. V. Siomoupoulis, "Is Mania Over-Diagnosed?" *Behavioral Medicine* (March 1981): 21.

46. Ibid.

47. Robert Seidenberg and Karen DeCrow, *Women Who Marry Houses: Panic and Protest in Agoraphobia,* (New York: McGraw-Hill, 1983), p. 127.

48. Snyder, p. 253.

Chapter 8. Involuntary Psychiatry and the Rule of Law

1. For a historical review of the laws, see George Rosen, *Madness and Society* (New York: Harper Torchbooks, 1969). See also Michel Foucault, *Madness and Civilization* (New York: Vintage Books, 1973).

2. Nicholas Kittrie, *The Right to Be Different: Deviance and Enforced Therapy* (Baltimore: Johns Hopkins Press, 1971), pp. 8–11.

3. Erving Goffman's *Asylums* (Garden City, N.Y.: Anchor Books, 1961) is the classic work on the nature of "total institutions" like prisons and mental hospitals.

4. For the incredible variety of abuses foisted on patients, and labeled as treatment, see Richard Hunter and Ida MacAlpine, *Three Hundred Years of Psychiatry* (London: Oxford University Press, 1963).

5. See, for example, U.S. Congress, Senate, Committee on the Judiciary, Subcommittee on Constitutional Rights, *Constitutional Rights of the Mentally Ill,* 87th Cong., 1st sess., 1961.

6. Alan Stone, *Mental Health and Law: A System in Transition,* Publication no. 76-176 (Washington, D.C.: Department of Health, Education, and Welfare, 1975), p. 46.

7. *Donaldson v. O'Connor* 422 U.S. 563 (1975). For Donaldson's own account of his long incarceration and battle to regain his freedom, see Kenneth Donaldson, *Insanity Inside Out* (New York: Crown, 1976).

8. *Baxstrom v. Herold* 383 U.S. 107 (1966).

9. For a summary of these developments, see John Monahan, "The Prevention of Violence," in John Monahan, ed., *Community Mental Health and the Criminal Justice System* (New York: Pergamon, 1975), p. 13.

10. See Introduction, n. 1.

11. *Tarasoff v. Regents of University of California* 13 Cal. 3d 425 (1976).

12. American Psychiatric Association, *amicus curiae* brief, *Tarasoff v. Regents of University of California* 551 P.2d 334 (1976).

13. Stone, p. 69.

14. Ibid., p. 67.

15. Loren Roth, "A Commitment Law for Patients, Doctors, and Lawyers," *American Journal of Psychiatry* 136 (1979): 1121.

16. Carol Warren, "Involuntary Commitment for Mental Disorder: The Application of California's Lanterman-Petris-Short Act," *Law and Society Review* 11 (1977): 629.

17. Supreme Court Study Commission on the Mentally Disabled and the Courts, "Civil Commitment in Minnesota," *Hamline Law Review* 4 (August 1980): 1.

18. Doug Cameron, *How to Survive Being Committed to a Mental Hospital* (New York: Vantage, 1979), p. 4.

19. Ibid., p. 8.

20. Ibid., p. 11.

21. Ibid., p. 17.

22. The following two examples, of "Nan" and "Bill," are taken from the medical records sent to me by each of the individuals involved. All quotations are taken directly from the medical records.

23. See *Hawaii Health Code,* chap. 334.

24. *Coleman v. Hart*, Superior Court, Alameda County, California, No. 482350-0, *Memorandum of Points and Authorities in Support of Plaintiff's Motion for Summary Judgment or for Adjudication of Issues without Substantial Controversy or for Preliminary Injunctive Relief*, Department 19 (June 3, 1980): 30.
25. Ibid., p. 34.
26. Ibid.
27. Ibid., p. 36.
28. Grant Morris, "Conservatorship for the 'Gravely Disabled': California's Nondeclaration of Nonindependence," *International Journal of Law and Psychiatry* 1 (1978): 395.
29. Ibid., p. 416.
30. Ibid.
31. Ibid., pp. 417–418.
32. Ibid., p. 420. Morris also cites an independent study that corroborates his findings. See B. Elliott, et al., "Conservatorship in San Diego County, 1974–1975: An Exploratory Descriptive Study of Conservatees and Placement Process" (Master's thesis, San Diego State University School of Social Work, 1976).
33. Morris, pp. 422–423.
34. Ibid., p. 423.
35. Ibid., p. 418.
36. California Senate Rules Committee and Board of Supervisors of San Diego County, *Report of a Joint Venture: A Comprehensive Review of Tax-Supported Health Services in San Diego County* 57 (Sacramento, California Senate Rules Committee, 1975), p. 62.
37. Cited as "Statement of David Owens, M.D., to San Diego Mental Health Association Task Force on Conservatorships, Feb. 17, 1975" (Morris, p. 419, n. 173).
38. D. Phillips, "Rejection: A Possible Consequence of Seeking Help for Mental Disorders," *American Sociological Review* 28 (1963): 963. See also J. Tringo, "The Hierarchy of Preference toward Disability Groups," *Journal of Special Education* (Summer 1970): 295.

Chapter 9. Abolishing Involuntary Treatment

1. See G. Gulevich and P. Bourne, "Mental Illness and Violence," in D. Daniels, M. Gilula, and F. Ochberg, eds., *Violence and the Struggle for Existence* (Boston: Little, Brown, 1970). Gulevich

and Bourne conclude their review by commenting, "An individual with a label of mental illness is quite capable of committing any act of violence known to man, but probably does not do so with any greater frequency than his neighbor in the general population" (p. 323).

2. *Time*, October 18, 1982, p. 18.

3. Lee Coleman, "Perspectives on the Medical Research of Violence," *American Journal of Orthopsychiatry* 44 (October 1974): 675.

4. Saleem Shah, "Dangerousness and Civil Commitment of the Mentally Ill: Some Public Policy Considerations," *American Journal of Psychiatry* 132 (May 1975): 503.

5. One indication of our inability to reduce the incidence of suicide through forced treatment is the fact that in cities with suicide prevention centers the suicide rate is as high as the rate in cities without centers. See David Lester, "Effect of Suicide Prevention Centers on Suicide Rate in the United States," *Health Service Reports* 89 (January-February 1974): 37. Lester writes that "suicide prevention centers do not appear to have a statistically significant effect on the suicide rates of cities" (p. 38). He concludes that "we must view with some concern the relative immunity of suicide rates in the United States, despite the efforts of suicide prevention centers to decrease these rates. It may well be that suicide prevention centers do not prevent suicide." See also David Lester, "The Myth of Suicide Prevention," *Comprehensive Psychiatry* 13 (1972): 555.

6. David Greenberg, "Involuntary Psychiatric Commitments to Prevent Suicide," *New York University Law Review* 49 (1974): 256. See also Kent Miller, *Managing Madness: The Case Against Civil Commitment* (New York: Free Press, 1976), pp. 69-72.

7. Greenberg, p. 258.

8. Peter Breggin, *Psychiatric Drugs: Hazards to the Brain* (New York: Springer, 1983), p. 268.

9. Ibid.

10. Thomas Szasz, *Law, Liberty, and Psychiatry* (New York: Collier, 1963), p. 227.

11. T. Gutheil, "Editorial: In Search of True Freedom: Drug Refusal, Involuntary Medication, and 'Rotting with Your Rights On,'" *American Journal of Psychiatry* 137 (March 1980): 327.

12. Alan Stone, *Mental Health and Law: A System in Transition*, Publication no. 76-176 (Washington, D.C.: Department of Health, Education, and Welfare, 1975), p. 48.

13. For an excellent account of the lawlessness that allows the conservatorship process to be so readily invoked, see Grant Morris, "Conservatorship for the 'Gravely Disabled': California's Nondeclaration of Nonindependence," *International Journal of Law and Psychiatry* 1 (1978): 395.

14. Ronald Goldfarb, *Jails: The Ultimate Ghetto of the Criminal Justice System* (Garden City, N.Y.: Anchor Books, 1976).

15. See Goldfarb, chap. 3, for a discussion of the inadequate treatment resources available to jail inmates.

16. See Robert Mendelsohn, *Confessions of a Medical Heretic* (New York: Warner Books, 1979). Mendelsohn comments on the difficulty patients often have in receiving adequate information from their doctors: "You have to sit down and decide whether or not you want to take the drug. Again, don't trust your doctor's decision. Even if you can get him to admit to the side effects, he'll most likely discount them by saying they occur only in a small percentage of cases" (p. 83).

17. See, for example, Loren Roth, "A Commitment Law for Patients, Doctors, and Lawyers," *American Journal of Psychiatry* 136 (1979): 1121. Roth argues that "laws . . . have always permitted substitute permission for treatment of medical patients who are demonstrated incompetent to consent or refuse treatment. This is the medical model of mental health commitment" (p. 1122).

18. Judi Chamberlin, *On Our Own: Patient-Controlled Alternatives to the Mental Health System* (New York: Hawthorne, 1978), p. 111.

Chapter 10. The Crime of Treatment

1. See generally, Jessica Mitford, *Kind and Usual Punishment: The Prison Business* (New York: Vintage, 1974).

2. There is now a large literature dealing with these developments. Particularly useful are David Rothman, *The Discovery of the Asylum: Social Order and Disorder in the New Republic* (Boston: Little, Brown, 1971), and Michel Foucault, *Discipline and Punish: The Birth of the Prison* (New York: Pantheon, 1977).

3. *In re Rodriguez* 14 Cal. 3d 639 (1975), p. 643.

4. Ibid.

5. Ibid., n. 16.

6. For a brief but cogent discussion of this capriciousness, see American Friends Service Committee, *Struggle for Justice: A Report on Crime and Punishment in America* (New York: Hill and Wang, 1971).

7. See the works by Rothman and Foucault (cited in n. 2).

8. Gustav Aschaffenburg, *Crime and Its Repression* (Boston: Little, Brown, 1913), pp. vi–vii.

9. George Ives, *A History of Penal Methods* (London: Stanley Paul, 1914), p. 335.

10. Ernest Hoag and Edward Williams, *Crime, Abnormal Minds, and the Law* (Indianapolis: Bobbs-Merrill, 1923), p. xiii.

11. Harry Barnes and Negley Teeters, *New Horizons in Criminology* (New York: Prentice-Hall, 1951), pp. 817–818.

12. Ibid., p. xviii.

13. James McConnell, "Criminals Can Be Brainwashed—NOW," *Psychology Today*, April 1970, p. 74.

14. Edward Opton, "Psychiatric Violence against Prisoners: When Therapy Is Punishment," *Mississippi Law Journal* 45 (1974): 605; Wayne Sage, "Crime and the Clockwork Lemon," *Human Behavior* (September 1974): 16; Stephen Sansweet, "Aversion Therapy: Punishing of People to Change Behavior Gains Use, Controversy," *Wall Street Journal*, January 2, 1974, p. 1; Stephen Sansweet, *The Punishment Cure* (New York: Mason-Charter, 1975). A primary source of documentation is U.S. Congress, Senate, Committee on the Judiciary, Subcommittee on Constitutional Rights, *Individual Rights and the Federal Role in Behavior Modification*, 93d Cong., 2d sess., 1974.

15. G. Livingston, *Exiles End* (London: Lyrebird Press, 1973), pp. 101–102.

16. Robert Martinson, "What Works—Questions and Answers about Prison Reform," *The Public Interest* 35 (Spring 1974): 22.

17. See, for example, Henry Steadman, "The Psychiatrist as a Conservative Agent of Social Control," *Social Problems* 20 (Fall 1972): 266.

18. Paul Dickson, "The Inmate Press," *The Nation*, April 27, 1974, p. 527.

19. Alfred Hassan, "The Pit," in Eve Pell, ed., *Maximum Security: Letters from Prison* (New York: Dutton, 1972), p. 28.

20. Ibid., p. 31.

21. Ibid., p. 32.

22. Ibid.
23. From a personal letter written in 1972 by a California state prisoner to the Committee for Prisoner Humanity and Justice, San Rafael, California.
24. Foucault, p. 10.
25. A good discussion of why punishment is preferable to treatment can be found in Herbert Morris, "Persons and Punishment," *The Monist* 52 (1968): 475. Morris unfortunately fails to see that coercive "treatment" is just as destructive to mental patients as to prisoners. For more on the nature of criminal punishment, see Rudolph Gerber and Patrick McAnany, eds., *Contemporary Punishment: Views, Explanations, and Justifications* (Notre Dame, Ind.: University of Notre Dame, 1972); Ernest van den Haag, *Punishing Criminals* (New York: Basic Books, 1975); Hyman Gross and Andrew von Hirsch, *Sentencing* (New York: Oxford University Press, 1981); Andrew von Hirsch, *Doing Justice: The Choice of Punishments* (New York: Hill and Wang, 1976). See also chapter 7 of American Friends Service Committee, *Struggle for Justice.*
26. Examples of the impact of uncertainty are not hard to find. A frequent statement made by the families of American embassy employees interned in Iran was that the uncertainty—not the separation—was the most difficult part of their ordeal. Families of Vietnam MIAs voiced similar feelings.
27. A typical example, from clinical work with psychotherapy patients, is the fact that marital counseling usually fails unless *both* persons are motivated for therapy. When one person (usually the woman) pressures the other to initiate joint counseling, little progress occurs. Real therapy requires a very personal commitment to the process. In or out of prison, personal decisions cannot be mandated by others.
28. See American Friends Service Committee, cited in n. 6.
29. Some authorities have suggested that sentencing commissions—perhaps appointed by state legislatures—would be better suited to perform this function. See, for example, M. Frankel, *Criminal Sentences* (New York: Hill and Wang, 1972), chap. 9. See also M. Tonry, "The Sentencing Commission in Sentencing Reform," *Hofstra Law Review* 7 (1979): 315, and J. Coffee, "The Repressed Issues in Sentencing: Accountability, Predictability, and Equality in the Era of the Sentencing Commission," *Georgetown Law Review* 66 (1978): 975. However sentences are determined, by the legislatures or by sentencing commissions, the main point

is for a sentence to reflect the harm done by the crime, not the criminal's "mental health" or "dangerousness." For more details on the California system, see A. Cassou and B. Taugher, "Determinate Sentencing in California: The New Numbers Game," *Pacific Law Journal* 9 (1978): 5. See also S. Messinger and P. Johnson, "California's Determinate Sentencing Statute: History and Issues," in National Institute of Law Enforcement and Criminal Justice, *Determinate Sentencing: Reform or Regression?* (Washington, D.C.: U.S. Government Printing Office, 1978), pp. 13-58.

30. According to a summary prepared by the National Council on Crime and Delinquency, Research Center, 760 Market St., San Francisco, California, 94102, thirteen states passed some form of determinate sentencing legislation in the period 1977-1980. None, however, mandates the degree of determinacy I have proposed. For the latest information on the current status of sentencing legislation, the reader is referred to the Criminal Courts Technical Assistance Project, Institute for Advanced Studies in Justice, Washington College of Law, The American University, Washington, D.C.

31. The thorny problem of codification of sentences is discussed in Gross and von Hirsch, pp. 303-335. Guidelines for judges are discussed in Don Gottfredson, Leslie Wilkins, and Peter Hoffman, *Guidelines for Parole and Sentencing: A Policy Control Method* (Lexington, Mass.: Lexington Books, 1978). See also Leslie Wilkins, et al., *Sentencing Guidelines: Structuring Judicial Discretion* (Washington, D.C.: U.S. Government Printing Office, 1978). For further information on "presumptive sentencing," in which the legislatures (or commissions established by them) determine sentences that may be only slightly altered by the trial judge, see Twentieth Century Fund, *Fair and Certain Punishment: Report of the Twentieth Century Fund Task Force on Criminal Sentencing* (New York: McGraw-Hill, 1976), as well as von Hirsch, *Doing Justice;* David Fogel and Joe Hudson, *Justice as Fairness: Perspectives on the Justice Model* (Cincinnati: Anderson, 1981). See also Richard Singer, *Just Deserts: Sentencing Based on Equality and Desert* (Cambridge, Mass.: Ballinger, 1979).

32. The Committee for the Study of Incarceration, Charles Goodell, chairman, has reached conclusions about sentencing reform similar to mine. Regarding alternatives to incarceration, the committee stated, "Today's prisons and jails are populated not only by murderers and muggers but also by marijuana offenders,

prostitutes, pickpockets, writers of bad checks and car thieves. Under our conception, less severe alternative punishments will have to be devised for the not-so-serious offenders that constitute the bulk of the system's caseload." The committee's report has been published as *Doing Justice*, by Andrew von Hirsch; for the quotation see page 118.

33. See American Friends Service Committee (cited in n. 6), pp. 83-99.

34. For a brief summary of these studies, see Howard Sachs and Charles Logan, *Does Parole Make a Difference?* (Hartford: University of Connecticut School of Law Press, 1979), pp. 67-71. They conclude that existing studies of parole are "inconclusive as to the efficacy of parole in an American state system." To my knowledge, there are no studies that test the proposal that discharged prisoners be free of mandatory parole surveillance, yet be provided with voluntary postrelease services. Such a study would be easy to accomplish, inexpensive, and without risk to society.

35. The American Bar Association's Committee on the Legal Status of Prisoners has also made this recommendation. They write, "On the date of release . . . the prisoner should be released from confinement without further conditions or supervision. The correctional authority should provide counselling and other assistance to released prisoners on a voluntary basis for at least one year after release." See American Bar Association Committee on the Legal Status of Prisoners, "Tentative Draft of Standards Relating to the Legal Status of Prisoners," *American Criminal Law Review* 14 (1977): 606-608.

Chapter 11. Children and the Double Standard of Justice

1. For a summary of the workings of the juvenile court, see Nicholas Kittrie, *The Right to Be Different: Deviance and Enforced Therapy* (Baltimore: Johns Hopkins Press, 1971), chap. 3.

2. Anthony Platt, *The Child Savers: The Invention of Delinquency* (Chicago: University of Chicago Press, 1969). See also Sanford Fox, "Juvenile Justice Reform: An Historical Perspective," *Stanford Law Review* 22 (June 1970): 1187. Fox makes the important point in this thorough review of the nineteenth-century predecessors of the juvenile court system, that the new Illinois Juvenile Court founded in 1899 was neither as benevolent as its rhetoric implied nor as innovative as most later historians believed. See also Steven Schlossman, *Love and the American*

Delinquent: The Theory and Practice of Progressive Juvenile Justice, 1825–1920 (Chicago: University of Chicago Press, 1977).

3. See, for example, Daniel Katkin, "Children and the Justice Process: Reality and Rhetoric," in David Gottlieb, ed., *Children's Liberation* (Englewood Cliffs, N.J.: Prentice-Hall, 1973); Patrick Murphy, *Our Kindly Parent . . . the State* (New York: Viking, 1974); Charles Silberman, *Criminal Violence, Criminal Justice* (New York: Vintage, 1980), chap. 9; Frances Allen, *The Borderland of Criminal Justice* (Chicago: University of Chicago Press, 1964), pp. 43–61.

4. Quoted in Silberman, p. 419.

5. Billie Holiday, *Lady Sings the Blues* (New York: Lancer Books, 1969), pp. 16–17.

6. *In re Gault* 387 U.S. 1 (1967).

7. See Aryeh Neier, *Crime and Punishment: A Radical Solution* (New York: Scarborough Books, 1978), chap. 8.

8. For writings on juvenile incarceration, see Kenneth Wooden, *Weeping in the Playtime of Others: America's Incarcerated Children* (New York: McGraw-Hill, 1976); Larry Cole, *Our Children's Keepers: Inside America's Kid Prisons* (Greenwich, Conn.: Fawcett Premier, 1972); Howard James, *Children in Trouble: A National Scandal* (New York: Pocket Books, 1971); Edward Wakin, *Children without Justice* (New York: National Council of Jewish Women, 1975); Thomas J. Cottle, *Children in Jail: Seven Lessons in American Justice* (Boston: Beacon Press, 1977).

9. Celeste McLeod, "Street Girls of the Seventies," *The Nation*, April 20, 1974, p. 487.

10. This is the figure given by Neier on page 94, as of 1975. Wakin estimates the total number of yearly juvenile arrests, for all offenses, at more than two million (p. 11).

11. Neier, p. 95.

12. Meda Chesney-Lind, "Young Women in the Arms of the Law: An Inquiry into the Treatment of Female Delinquents in the Juvenile Justice System," in Ruth Crow and Ginny McCarthy, eds., *Teenage Women in the Juvenile Justice System: Changing Values* (Tucson, Ariz.: New Directions for Young Women, 1979), p. 53.

13. Ibid., p. 56.

14. Silberman, pp. 421–422.

15. Chesney-Lind, p. 57.

16. Ibid., pp. 59–61.
17. Richard Chused, "The Juvenile Court Process: A Study of Three New Jersey Counties," *Rutgers Law Review* 26 (1973): 507 and 509.
18. Ibid., pp. 523 and 529.
19. Chesney-Lind, p. 61.
20. Personal communication.
21. Nicholas Pileggi, "Inside the Juvenile Justice System: How Fifteen Year Olds Get Away with Murder," *New York*, June 13, 1977, p. 36.
22. Ibid., p. 41.
23. Ibid., p. 43.
24. Ibid.
25. Ibid.
26. Silberman, p. 424.
27. For a discussion of the lack of true expertise in child custody decisions, see Jay Ziskin, *Coping with Psychiatric and Psychological Testimony*, 3d ed. (Venice, Calif.: Law and Psychology Press, 1981), chap. 10. Ziskin comments that "such cases are heard by a judge rather than a jury. While many judges are open-minded concerning the capabilities of clinicians, there are many others who have a strong tendency to defer to their judgment." A careful reading of the accounts of even the most knowledgeable and circumspect of these "experts" will reveal that their skills as therapists do not help them in custody matters. Richard Gardner, associate clinical professor of psychiatry at the Columbia University College of Physicians and Surgeons, for example, writing in the July 24, 1979, issue of *Practicing Law Institute Newsletter*, states that "I am not particularly concerned with arriving at a final diagnosis. The court has asked my opinion regarding which parent would be the better one for the children. A diagnosis *per se* may not give any valid information in this regard." One may ask, then, why a doctor is needed if a diagnosis is unimportant. Gardner continues, "The most convincing reports are heavily weighted with direct quotations of statements made by the clients to the psychiatrist." Clearly, the transmission of direct quotes from parent to court hardly requires an "expert." Finally, Gardner concludes, "At the completion of my evaluation I review all materials and make a decision. I try to consider each parent's assets and liabilities regarding parental competence and decide which parent ends up with the best balance." This is exactly what the judge should be doing, but all

too often the psychiatrist's conclusions will be the determining factor.

28. See Boyd Dover, "Closing the Door to Status Offenders: One Juvenile Court's Experiment in Fairness and Equality," in Ruth Crow and Ginny McCarthy, eds., *Teenage Women in the Juvenile Justice System: Changing Values* (Tucson, Ariz.: New Directions for Young Women, 1979), p. 113. Dover, former director of Court Services for the Pima County Arizona Juvenile Court Center, proposes that we offer teen-age women the "right to receive services and to refuse services not viewed as useful or necessary" (p. 117).

29. Chesney-Lind, pp. 76–77.

30. This trend was prompted by the Juvenile Justice and Delinquency Prevention Act of 1974. Some states, like Massachusetts, California, and New York, now refuse to place "status offenders" in jail or in "training schools," but children are still forced to stay in group homes and foster homes. Frequently they are forced to engage in psychiatric therapy, whether they desire it or not. For further discussion of alternatives to our current method of dealing with youthful "status offenders," see Twentieth Century Fund, *Confronting Youth Crime: Report of the Twentieth Century Fund Task Force on Sentencing Policy toward Young Offenders* (New York: Holmes and Meier, 1978), and Robert D. Vintner, George Downs, and John Hall, *Juvenile Corrections in the States: Residential Programs and De-Institutionalization* (Ann Arbor, Mich.: National Assessment of Juvenile Corrections, University of Michigan, 1975).

31. David Bazelon, "Beyond Control of the Juvenile Court," *Juvenile Court Journal* 21 (Summer 1970): 44.

32. Silberman argues along similar lines: "Juveniles should not be incarcerated, or their liberty restricted in other ways, for the *purpose* of rehabilitation. But once the decision to punish a youngster has been made, there must be a serious attempt to provide whatever help he needs to become a productive member of society" (p. 483).

33. Sanford Fox, "The Reform of Juvenile Justice: The Child's Right to Punishment," *Juvenile Justice* 25 (August 1974): 4.

34. Ibid.

35. Ibid., p. 5.

36. Professor Fox has reached the same conclusion. "The matter of sentencing," he writes, "might rather be made to turn on the age of the child and the chronicity of his misconduct, as well as on the nature of his conduct" (ibid., p. 8).

SELECTED BIBLIOGRAPHY

Alexander, Shana. *Anyone's Daughter.* New York: Viking Press, 1979.

Allen, Frances. *The Borderland of Criminal Justice.* Chicago: University of Chicago Press, 1964.

American Friends Service Committee. *Struggle for Justice: A Report on Crime and Punishment in America.* New York: Hill and Wang, 1971.

American Psychiatric Association Insanity Defense Work Group. *Statement on the Insanity Defense.* Washington, D.C.: American Psychiatric Association, 1982.

American Psychiatric Association Task Force. *Electroconvulsive Therapy.* Report no. 14. Washington, D.C.: American Psychiatric Association, 1978.

———. "Tardive Dyskinesia: Summary of a Task Force Report of the American Psychiatric Association." *American Journal of Psychiatry* 137 (October 1980): 1163.

Anspacher, Carolyn. *The Trial of Dr. De Kaplany.* New York: Frederick Fell, 1965.

Arenella, Peter. "The Diminished Capacity and Diminished Responsibility Defenses: Two Children of a Doomed Marriage." *Columbia Law Review* 77 (October 1977): 827.

Aschaffenburg, Gustav. *Crime and Its Repression.* Boston: Little, Brown, 1913.

Ayd, Frank. "The Depot Fluphenazines: A Reappraisal after Ten Years' Clinical Experience." *American Journal of Psychiatry* 132 (May 1975): 491.

Balter, Mitchell, and Bauer, Mary Lou. "Patterns of Prescribing and Use of Hypnotic Drugs in the United States." In A. D. Clift, ed., *Sleep Disturbance and Hypnotic Drug Dependence.* Amsterdam: Excerpta Medica, 1975.

Barnes, Harry, and Teeters, Negley. *New Horizons in Criminology.* New York: Prentice-Hall, 1951.

Bazelon, David. "Beyond Control of the Juvenile Court." *Juvenile Court Journal* 21 (Summer 1970): 44.

Bowart, Walter. *Operation Mind Control.* New York: Dell, 1978.

Breggin, Peter. "Coercion of Voluntary Patients in an Open Hospital." *Archives of General Psychiatry* 10 (February 1964): 173.

———. *Electroshock: Its Brain-Disabling Effects.* New York: Springer, 1979.

———. "Psychiatry and the CIA Connection." *Libertarian Review* (September 1979): 32.

———. "Brain-Disabling Therapies." In Elliot Valenstein, ed., *The Psychosurgery Debate: Scientific, Legal, and Ethical Perspectives.* San Francisco: W. H. Freeman, 1980.

———. *Psychiatric Drugs: Hazards to the Brain.* New York: Springer, 1983.

Brooks, Alexander. *Law, Psychiatry, and the Mental Health System.* Boston: Little, Brown, 1974.

Bryant, Robert Park, and Hume, Corbin Brooke. "Diminished Capacity—Recent Decisions and an Analytic Approach." *Vanderbilt Law Review* 30 (1977): 213.

Caligari, Dr. [Richman, David]. "From Guinea Pig to Guinea Pig." *Madness Network News* 3 (December 1975): 11.

———. "Psychiatric Drug Deaths." *On the Edge: Newsletter of the Bay Area Committee For Alternatives to Psychiatry* 2 (June 1981): 3.

Cameron, Doug. *How to Survive Being Committed to a Mental Hospital.* New York: Vantage, 1979.

Cameron, D. Ewen; Lohrenz, J. G.; and Handcock, K. A. "The Depatterning Treatment of Schizophrenia." *Comprehensive Psychiatry* 3 (April 1962): 65.

Cassou, A., and Taugher, B. "Determinate Sentencing in California: The New Numbers Game." *Pacific Law Journal* 9 (1978): 5.

Chamberlin, Judi. *On Our Own: Patient-Controlled Alternatives to the Mental Health System.* New York: Hawthorne, 1978.

Chandler, Daniel, and Sallychild, Andrea. *The Use and Misuse of Psychiatric Drugs in California's Mental Health Programs,* no. 31. Sacramento: Assembly Office of Research, June 1977.

Chesney-Lind, Meda. "Young Women in the Arms of the Law: An Inquiry into the Treatment of Female Delinquents in the Juvenile Justice System." In Ruth Crow and Ginny McCarthy, eds., *Teenage Women in the Juvenile Justice System: Changing Values.* Tucson, Ariz.: New Directions for Young Women, 1979.

Chiong, Boo. "The Evidence against the Catecholamine Hypothesis." *Psychiatric Opinion* (September 1979): 10.

Chu, Franklin, and Trotter, Sharland. *The Madness Establishment.* New York: Grossman, 1974.

Chused, Richard. "The Juvenile Court Process: A Study of Three New Jersey Counties." *Rutgers Law Review* 26 (1973): 488.

Coffee, J. "The Repressed Issues in Sentencing: Accountability, Predictability, and Equality in the Era of the Sentencing Commission." *Georgetown Law Review* 66 (1978): 975.

Cole, Larry. *Our Children's Keepers: Inside America's Kid Prisons.* Greenwich, Conn.: Fawcett Premier, 1972.

Coleman, Lee. "Perspectives on the Medical Research of Violence." *American Journal of Orthopsychiatry* 44 (October 1974): 675.

————. "Problem Kids and Preventive Medicine: The Making of an Odd Couple." *American Journal of Orthopsychiatry* 48 (January 1978): 56.

Cottle, Thomas J. *Children in Jail: Seven Lessons in American Justice.* Boston: Beacon Press, 1977.

Crane, George. "Clinical Psychopharmacology in Its Twentieth Year." *Science* 181 (July 13, 1973): 124.

Davis, John. "Overview: Maintenance Therapy in Psychiatry: I. Schizophrenia." *American Journal of Psychiatry* 132 (December 1975): 1237.

Delgado-Escueta, Antonio V., et al. "Special Report: The Nature of Aggression during Epileptic Seizures." *New England Journal of Medicine* 305 (September 17, 1981): 711.

Diamond, Bernard. "Isaac Ray and the Trial of Daniel M'Naughten." *American Journal of Psychiatry* 112 (February 1956): 651.

————. "Criminal Responsibility of the Mentally Ill." *Stanford Law Review* 14 (1961): 59.

Dickson, Paul. "The Inmate Press." *The Nation,* April 27, 1974, p. 527.

Donaldson, Kenneth. *Insanity Inside Out.* New York: Crown, 1976.

Dover, Boyd. "Closing the Door to Status Offenders: One Juvenile Court's Experiment in Fairness and Equality." In Ruth Crow and Ginny McCarthy, eds., *Teenage Women in the Juvenile Justice System: Changing Values.* Tucson, Ariz.: New Directions for Young Women, 1979.

Ennis, Bruce. *Prisoners of Psychiatry.* New York: Avon Books, 1972.

Ennis, Bruce, and Litwack, Thomas. "Psychiatry and the Presumption of Expertise." *California Law Review* 62 (May 1974): 693.

Fersch, Ellsworth. *Psychology and Psychiatry in Courts and Corrections.* New York: Wiley-Interscience, 1980.

Fieve, Ronald. *Moodswing: The Third Revolution in Psychiatry.* New York: William Morrow, 1975.

Fogel, David, and Hudson, Joe. *Justice as Fairness: Perspectives on the Justice Model.* Cincinnati: Anderson, 1981.

Foucault, Michel. *Madness and Civilization.* New York: Vintage Books, 1973.

———. *Discipline and Punish: The Birth of the Prison.* New York: Pantheon, 1977.

Fox, Sanford. "Juvenile Justice Reform: An Historical Perspective." *Stanford Law Review* 22 (June 1970): 1187.

———. "The Reform of Juvenile Justice: The Child's Right to Punishment." *Juvenile Justice* 25 (August 1974): 2.

Frank, Leonard, ed. *The History of Shock Treatment.* Mr. Frank, 2300 Webster St., San Francisco, Calif. 94115, 1978.

Frankel, M. *Criminal Sentences.* New York: Hill and Wang, 1972.

Freedman, Alfred, and Kaplan, Harold, eds. *Comprehensive Textbook of Psychiatry.* Baltimore: Williams and Wilkins, 1967.

Freeman, Walter; Watts, James; and Hunt, Thelma. *Psychosurgery: Intelligence, Emotion, and Social Behavior following Prefrontal Lobotomy for Mental Disorders.* Springfield, Ill.: Charles C Thomas, 1942.

Friedberg, John. "Shock Treatment, Brain Damage, and Memory Loss: A Neurological Perspective." *American Journal of Psychiatry* 134 (September 1977): 1010.

Fulgoni, Dino. "Medieval Systematics in the Modern Law of Crime." *Prosecutor's Brief: Journal of the California District Attorneys Association* 3 (January–February 1980): 10.

Gardos, George, and Cole, Jonathan. "Maintenance Antipsychotic Therapy: Is the Cure Worse Than the Disease?" *American Journal of Psychiatry* 133 (January 1976): 32.

Gerber, Rudolph, and McAnany, Patrick, eds. *Contemporary Punishment: Views, Explanations, and Justifications.* Notre Dame, Ind.: University of Notre Dame, 1972.

Goffman, Erving. *Asylums.* Garden City, N.Y.: Anchor Books, 1961.

Goldfarb, Ronald. *Jails: The Ultimate Ghetto of the Criminal Justice System.* Garden City, N.Y.: Anchor Books, 1976.

Goodwin, Frederick. "Introduction to the Lithium Ion." *Archives of General Psychiatry* 36 (July 1979): 834.

Gorman, Mike. *Every Other Bed.* Cleveland, Oh.: World, 1956.

Goshen, Charles, ed. *Documentary History of Psychiatry.* New York: Philosophical Library, 1967.

Gottfredson, Don; Wilkins, Leslie; and Hoffman, Peter. *Guidelines for Parole and Sentencing: A Policy Control Method.* Lexington, Mass.: Lexington Books, 1978.

Greenberg, David. "Involuntary Psychiatric Commitments to Prevent Suicide." *New York University Law Review* 49 (1974): 227.

Gross, Hyman, and von Hirsch, Andrew. *Sentencing.* New York: Oxford University Press, 1981.

Group for the Advancement of Psychiatry. *Misuse of Psychiatry in the Criminal Courts: Competency to Stand Trial.* Vol. 8, Report no. 89. New York: Group for the Advancement of Psychiatry, 1974.

Gulevich, G., and Bourne, P. "Mental Illness and Violence." In D. Daniels, M. Gilula, and F. Ochberg, eds., *Violence and the Struggle for Existence.* Boston: Little, Brown, 1970.

Gutheil, T. "Editorial: In Search of True Freedom: Drug Refusal, Involuntary Medication, and 'Rotting with Your Rights On.'" *American Journal of Psychiatry* 137 (March 1980): 327.

Halpern, Abraham. "Use and Misuse of Psychiatry in Competency Examinations of Criminal Defendants." *Psychiatric Annals* 5.4 (April 1975): 8.

Harris, T. George. "Psychiatrist Bernard L. Diamond Tells of the Bizarre Paranoia He Found in Sirhan B. Sirhan: A Conversation with T. George Harris." *Psychology Today,* September 1969, p. 48.

Hassan, Alfred. "The Pit." In Eve Pell, ed., *Maximum Security: Letters from Prison.* New York: Dutton, 1972.

Hinckle, Warren. "Dan White's San Francisco." *Inquiry,* October 29, 1979, p. 8.

Hoag, Ernest, and Williams, Edward. *Crime, Abnormal Minds, and the Law.* Indianapolis: Bobbs-Merrill, 1923.

Hoch, Paul. "Experimentally Produced Psychoses." *American Journal of Psychiatry* 107 (February 1951): 607.

Holiday, Billie. *Lady Sings the Blues.* New York: Lancer Books, 1969.

Hughes, Richard, and Brewin, Robert. *The Tranquilizing of America.* New York: Harcourt Brace Jovanovich, 1979.

Hunter, Richard, and MacAlpine, Ida. *Three Hundred Years of Psychiatry: 1535-1860.* London: Oxford University Press, 1963.

Illich, Ivan. *Medical Nemesis: The Expropriation of Health.* New York: Random House, 1976.

Ives, George. *A History of Penal Methods.* London: Stanley Paul, 1914.

Jackson, George. *Soledad Brother: The Prison Letters of George Jackson.* New York: Bantam Books, 1970.

James, Howard. *Children in Trouble: A National Scandal.* New York: Pocket Books, 1971.

Jenner, Frederick. "Lithium and the Question of Kidney Damage." *Archives of General Psychiatry* 36 (July 1979): 888.

Johnson, Phillip E. "The Supreme Court of California, 1975–1976: Foreword—The Accidental Decision and How It Happens." *California Law Review* 65 (1977): 231.

Kahn, Howard, and Porter, Martin. "The Secret Army Drug Experiments: What Did Warren Burger Know?" *Rolling Stone*, April 21, 1977, p. 46.

Kalinowsky, Lothar. "The Convulsive Therapies." In Alfred Freedman, Harold Kaplan, and Benjamin Sadock, eds., *Comprehensive Textbook of Psychiatry*, 2d ed. Baltimore: Williams and Wilkins, 1975.

Katkin, Daniel. "Children and the Justice Process: Reality and Rhetoric." In David Gottlieb, ed., *Children's Liberation*. Englewood Cliffs, N.J.: Prentice-Hall, 1973.

Kittrie, Nicholas. *The Right to Be Different: Deviance and Enforced Therapy*. Baltimore: Johns Hopkins Press, 1971.

Latz, John, and Jenkins, Gaye. "Lithium: Miracle Drug or Emotional Straitjacket?" *State and Mind* (Spring 1978): 25.

Lawler, James. *I.Q., Heritability, and Racism*. New York: International Publishers, 1978.

Lehmann, H. "The Philosophy of Long Acting Medication in Psychiatry." *Diseases of the Nervous System* 31 Supp. (September 1970): 7.

Lennard, Henry; Epstein, Leon; Bernstein, Arnold; and Ransom, Donald. *Mystification and Drug Misuse*. New York: Perennial Library, 1971.

Lester, David. "The Myth of Suicide Prevention." *Comprehensive Psychiatry* 13 (1972): 555.

———. "Effect of Suicide Prevention Centers on Suicide Rate in the United States." *Health Service Reports* 89 (January-February 1974): 37.

Lewis, Nolan D., and Strahl, Margaret O., eds. *The Complete Psychiatrist: The Achievements of Paul H. Hoch, M.D.* Albany: State University of New York Press, 1968.

Lipp, Martin. *The Bitter Pill: Doctors, Patients, and Failed Expectations*. New York: Harper and Row, 1980.

Livingston, G. *Exiles End*. London: Lyrebird Press, 1973.

Lunde, Donald. *Murder and Madness*. Stanford, Calif.: The Portable Stanford, 1975.

Markman, Allen. "Death by Psychiatry: A Preliminary Review of Eight Deaths in the New York State Psychiatric System." *Phoenix Rising* 3 (Spring 1983): 5.

Marks, John. *The Search for the Manchurian Candidate: The CIA and Mind Control*. New York: New York Times Books, 1979.

Martinson, Robert. "What Works—Questions and Answers about Prison Reform." *The Public Interest* 35 (Spring 1974): 22.

McConnell, James. "Criminals Can Be Brainwashed—NOW." *Psychology Today*, April 1970, p. 14.

McGarry, Louis. "Demonstration and Research in Competency for Trial and Mental Illness: Review and Preview." *Boston University Law Review* 49 (1969): 46.

McLeod, Celeste. "Street Girls of the Seventies." *The Nation*, April 20, 1974, p. 487.

Mendelsohn, Robert. *Confessions of a Medical Heretic.* New York: Warner Books, 1979.

Menninger, Karl. *The Crime of Punishment.* New York: Viking Press, 1966.

Messinger, S., and Johnson, P. "California's Determinate Sentencing Statute: History and Issues." In National Institute of Law Enforcement and Criminal Justice, *Determinate Sentencing: Reform or Regression?* Washington, D.C.: U.S. Government Printing Office, 1978.

Miller, Kent. *Managing Madness: The Case against Civil Commitment.* New York: Free Press, 1976.

Mitford, Jessica. *Kind and Usual Punishment: The Prison Business.* New York: Vintage, 1974.

Mollica, Richard F. "From Asylum to Community: The Threatened Disintegration of Public Psychiatry." *New England Journal of Medicine* 308 (February 17, 1983): 367.

Monahan, John. "The Prevention of Violence." In John Monahan, ed., *Community Mental Health and the Criminal Justice System.* New York: Pergamon, 1975.

Morris, Grant. "Conservatorship for the 'Gravely Disabled': California's Nondeclaration of Nonindependence." *International Journal of Law and Psychiatry* 1 (1978): 395.

Morris, Herbert. "Persons and Punishment." *The Monist* 52 (1968): 475.

Morse, Stephen J. "Crazy Behavior, Morals, and Science: An Analysis of Mental Health Law." *Southern California Law Review* 51 (May 1978): 527.

———. "Diminished Capacity: A Moral and Legal Conundrum." *International Journal of Law and Psychiatry* 2 (1979): 271.

Murphy, Patrick. *Our Kindly Parent . . . the State.* New York: Viking, 1974.

Neier, Aryeh. *Crime and Punishment: A Radical Solution.* New York: Scarborough Books, 1978.

Noble, June, and Noble, William. *The Psychiatric Fix: Psychiatry's Alarming Power over Our Lives.* New York: Delacorte, 1981.

Office of Planning and Program Analysis, California Department of Health. *Task Force Investigation of State Hospital Resident Deaths (1973-76).* Sacramento: California Department of Health, June 15, 1978.

Opton, Edward. "Psychiatric Violence against Prisoners: When Therapy Is Punishment." *Mississippi Law Journal* 45 (1974): 605.

Parker, Marjory. "California's New Scheme for the Commitment of Individuals Found Incompetent to Stand Trial." *Pacific Law Journal* 6 (July 1975): 484.

Phillips, D. "Rejection: A Possible Consequence of Seeking Help for Mental Disorders." *American Sociological Review* 28 (1963): 963.

Pileggi, Nicholas. "Inside the Juvenile Justice System: How Fifteen Year Olds Get Away with Murder." *New York,* June 13, 1977, p. 36.

Platt, Anthony. *The Child Savers: The Invention of Delinquency.* Chicago: University of Chicago Press, 1969.

Platt, Anthony, and Diamond, Bernard. "Origins of the 'Right and Wrong' Test of Criminal Responsibility and Its Subsequent Development in the United States: An Historical Survey." *California Law Review* 54 (1966): 1227.

Rappaport, Maurice; Hopkins, H. Kenneth; Hall, Karyl; Belleza, Teodoro; and Silverman, Julian. "Schizophrenics for Whom Phenothiazines May Be Contraindicated or Unnecessary." *International Pharmacopsychiatry* 13 (1978): 100.

Raskin, David. "Akathisia: A Side Effect to Be Remembered." *American Journal of Psychiatry* 129 (September 1972): 121.

Ray, Isaac. *A Treatise on the Medical Jurisprudence of Insanity.* Boston: Little, Brown, 1838.

Reisberg, Barry, and Gershon, Samuel. "Side Effects Associated with Lithium Therapy." *Archives of General Psychiatry* 36 (July 20, 1979): 879.

Rice, Marilyn. "The Rice Papers." In Leonard Frank, ed., *The History of Shock Treatment.* Mr. Frank, 2300 Webster St., San Francisco, Calif. 94115, 1978.

Rinkel, Max, and Himwich, Harold, eds. *Insulin Treatment in Psychiatry.* New York: Philosophical Library, 1959.

Robitscher, Jonas. *The Powers of Psychiatry.* Boston: Houghton Mifflin, 1980.

Roche, Philip. *The Criminal Mind.* New York: Grove Press, 1958.

Rogers, J. Maurice. "Drug Abuse—Just What the Doctor Ordered." *Psychology Today*, September 1971, p. 16.

Rosen, George. *Madness and Society.* New York: Harper Torchbooks, 1969.

Rosenhan, David. "On Being Sane in Insane Places." *Science* 179 (January 19, 1973): 250.

Roth, Loren. "A Commitment Law for Patients, Doctors, and Lawyers." *American Journal of Psychiatry* 136 (September 1979): 1121.

Rothman, David. *The Discovery of the Asylum: Social Order and Disorder in the New Republic.* Boston: Little, Brown, 1971.

Roueche, Berton. "As Empty as Eve." *The New Yorker*, September 9, 1974, p. 84.

Sachs, Howard, and Logan, Charles. *Does Parole Make a Difference?* Hartford: University of Connecticut School of Law Press, 1979.

Sackler, Arthur; Sackler, Mortimer; Sackler, Raymond; and Marti-Ibañez, Felix, eds. *The Great Physiodynamic Therapies in Psychiatry: An Historical Reappraisal.* New York: Hoeber-Harper, 1956.

Sage, Wayne. "Crime and the Clockwork Lemon." *Human Behavior* (September 1974): 16.

Sakel, Manfred. "The Classical Sakel Shock Treatment: A Reappraisal." In Arthur Sackler, Mortimer Sackler, Raymond Sackler, and Felix Marti-Ibañez, eds. *The Great Physiodynamic Therapies in Psychiatry: An Historical Reappraisal.* New York: Hoeber-Harper, 1956.

———. *Schizophrenia.* New York: Philosophical Library, 1958.

Sansweet, Stephen. *The Punishment Cure.* New York: Mason-Charter, 1975.

Scheflin, Alan, and Opton, Edward. *The Mind Manipulators.* New York: Paddington Press, 1978.

Schlossman, Steven. *Love and the American Delinquent: The Theory and Practice of Progressive Juvenile Justice, 1825-1920.* Chicago: University of Chicago Press, 1977.

Scull, Andrew. *Decarceration.* Englewood Cliffs, N.J.: Prentice-Hall, 1977.

Shader, Richard, and DiMascio, Alberto. *Psychotropic Drug Side Effects.* Baltimore: Williams and Wilkins, 1970.

Shah, Saleem. "Dangerousness and Civil Commitment of the Mentally Ill: Some Public Policy Considerations." *American Journal of Psychiatry* 132 (May 1974): 501.

Sheehan, Susan. "The Patient: Part I—Creedmoor Psychiatric Center." *The New Yorker*, May 25, 1979, p. 75.

Shutts, David. *Lobotomy: Resort to the Knife.* New York: Van Nostrand Reinhold, 1982.

Silberman, Charles. *Criminal Violence, Criminal Justice.* New York: Vintage, 1980.

Silverman, Milton, and Lee, Philip R. *Pills, Politics, and Profits.* Berkeley: University of California Press, 1974.

Singer, Anne. "Insanity Acquittals in the Seventies: Observations and Empirical Analysis of One Jurisdiction." *Mental Disability Law Reporter* 2 (1978): 406.

Singer, Richard. *Just Deserts: Sentencing Based on Equality and Desert.* Cambridge, Mass.: Ballinger, 1979.

Siomoupoulis, V. "Is Mania Over-Diagnosed?" *Behavioral Medicine* (March 1981): 21.

Slovenko, Ralph. *Psychiatry and Law.* Boston: Little, Brown, 1973.

Smith, Burke. "The Polygraph." *Scientific American* 216, no. 1 (January 1967): 25.

Snyder, Solomon. *Madness and the Brain.* New York: McGraw-Hill, 1974.

Steadman, Henry. "The Psychiatrist as a Conservative Agent of Social Control." *Social Problems* 20 (Fall 1972): 263.

———. *Beating a Rap? Defendants Found Incompetent to Stand Trial.* Chicago: University of Chicago Press, 1979.

———. "Insanity Acquittals in New York State, 1965-1978." *American Journal of Psychiatry* 137 (March 1980): 321.

Stebel, S. L. *The Shoe Leather Treatment.* Los Angeles: J. P. Tarcher/St. Martin's Press, 1980.

Steir, Charles, ed. *Blue Jolts: True Stories from the Cuckoo's Nest.* Washington, D.C.: New Republic Books, 1978.

Sterling, Peter. "Psychiatry's Drug Addiction." *The New Republic,* December 8, 1979, p. 14.

Stone, Alan. *Mental Health and Law: A System in Transition.* Publication no. 76-176. Washington, D.C.: Department of Health, Education, and Welfare, 1975.

Supreme Court Study Commission on the Mentally Disabled and the Courts. "Civil Commitment in Minnesota." *Hamline Law Review* 4 (August 1980): 1.

Szasz, Thomas. *Law, Liberty, and Psychiatry.* New York: Collier, 1963.

———. *Psychiatric Justice.* Westport, Conn.: Greenwood Press, 1965.

———. "Patriotic Poisoners." *The Humanist* (November-December 1976): 5.

Tobias, L. L., and MacDonald, M. L. "Withdrawal of Maintenance Drugs with Long-Term Hospitalized Patients: A Critical Review." *Psychological Bulletin* 81 (1974): 107.

Tonry, M. "The Sentencing Commission in Sentencing Reform." *Hofstra Law Review* 7 (1979): 315.

Tringo, J. "The Hierarchy of Preference toward Disability Groups." *Journal of Special Education* 4 (Summer 1970): 295.

Twentieth Century Fund. *Fair and Certain Punishment: Report of the Twentieth Century Fund Task Force on Criminal Sentencing.* New York: McGraw-Hill, 1976.

————. *Confronting Youth Crime: Report of the Twentieth Century Fund Task Force on Sentencing Policy toward Young Offenders.* New York: Holmes and Meier, 1978.

University of Pennsylvania Law Review Editors. "Comment: Commitment to Farview: Incompetency to Stand Trial." *University of Pennsylvania Law Review* 117 (1969): 1164.

U.S. Congress. Senate. Committee on the Judiciary. Subcommittee on Constitutional Rights. *Constitutional Rights of the Mentally Ill.* 87th Cong., 1st sess., 1961.

U.S. Congress. Senate. Committee on the Judiciary. Subcommittee on Constitutional Rights. *Individual Rights and the Federal Role in Behavior Modification.* 93d Cong., 2d sess., 1974.

Van Putten, Theodore. "Why Do Schizophrenic Patients Refuse to Take Their Drugs?" *Archives of General Psychiatry* 31 (July 1974): 67.

Vintner, Robert D.; Downs, George; and Hall, John. *Juvenile Corrections in the States: Residential Programs and De-Institutionalization.* Ann Arbor, Mich.: National Assessment of Juvenile Corrections, University of Michigan, 1975.

von Hirsch, Andrew. *Doing Justice: The Choice of Punishments.* New York: Hill and Wang, 1976.

Wakin, Edward. *Children without Justice.* New York: National Council of Jewish Women, 1975.

Waldron, Ingrid. "Increased Prescribing of Valium, Librium, and Other Drugs—An Example of the Influence of Economic and Social Factors on the Practice of Medicine." *International Journal of Health Services* 7 (1977): 37.

Walker, Nigel. *Crime and Insanity in England.* Edinburgh: Edinburgh University Press, 1968.

Warren, Carol. "Involuntary Commitment for Mental Disorder: The Application of California's Lanterman-Petris-Short Act." *Law and Society Review* 11 (1977): 629.

Wilkins, Leslie; Kress, J. M.; Gottfredson, Don; Calpin, J. C.; and Gelman, A. M. *Sentencing Guidelines: Structuring Judicial Discretion.* Washington, D.C.: U.S. Government Printing Office, 1978.

Winslade, William. *The Insanity Plea: The Uses and Abuses of the Insanity Defense.* New York: Charles Scribner's, 1983.

Wood, Jim. *The Rape of Inez Garcia.* New York: Putnam's, 1976.

Wooden, Kenneth. *Weeping in the Playtime of Others: America's Incarcerated Children.* New York: McGraw-Hill, 1976.

Ziskin, Jay. *Coping with Psychiatric and Psychological Testimony,* 3d ed. Venice, Calif.: Law and Psychology Press, 1981.

Zugibe, Frederick. "Sudden Death Related to the Use of Psychotropic Drugs." In Cyril H. Wecht, ed., *Legal Medicine, 1980.* Philadelphia: W. B. Saunders, 1980, p. 75.

INDEX

Lee Coleman, M.D., a practicing psychiatrist, is the founder and director of the Center for the Study of Psychiatric Testimony in Berkeley, California. An advisory board member of the Citizens Commission on Human Rights, which advances the rights of mental patients, he writes for both popular and professional journals on psychiatry and the law.